HOW TO USE TAI CHI FOR SELF-DEFENCE

7 Practical Steps to Develop Your Martial
Skills and Avoid Having to Use Them

by

Colin and Gaynel Hamilton

The 7 Steps Towards Mastery Series Volume 2

Disclaimer

The authors of this book are not responsible, in any manner whatsoever, for any damage or injury of any kind that may result from practicing or applying the principles, ideas or techniques described in this book.

As with any other type of unaccustomed exercise, readers are advised to consult a doctor before embarking on any kind of martial arts training.

ISBN: 9781980688938

For Jon Cooper

Acknowledgements

We would like to express our gratitude to all of our students, teachers and Tai Chi ancestors. In particular, we would like to thank our teachers: Dr. Zhu Guang, Robert France, Nigel Sutton, Ray Wilkie, Michael Tse and Dr. Chen Haifeng for their patient and inspired teaching and friendship; our Tai Chi Grandfather, Professor Wang Zhizhong; our training partners: Michael Stone, Mike Abosch, Mark Fahy, Ben Morris, Ben Bisco and Wu Zhe Ri, who have worked with us in the preservation and evolution of the martial aspects of our martial art - and Jon Cooper, a great police officer, dear friend and training partner for many years, who is sadly missed.

Special thanks also to Peter Consterdine and Geoff Thompson for their pioneering work in combining traditional martial arts with the realities of practical self-protection on the street, and for their kind permission to quote them on the main aims of the British Combat Association; to Barbara Doyle and Denis Penman, who have kindly proof-read our manuscript and provided helpful feedback during the production process; to Zoë Hamilton for her invaluable guidance on the cover design; to Jane Middleton for constantly prodding us to get on with it; to our many friends and fellow-instructors in the global Tai Chi community, including Bob Lowey, Ronnie Robinson, Chris Thomas, Dan Docherty, Eva and Karel Koskuba, Linda Broda, Marnix Wells and Gary Wragg; and, not least, to our thousands of students, past and present. We especially appreciate the tireless work of those who have gone on to become instructors in their own right, including Barbara Doyle, Kath Pybus, Mark Fahy, John Donegan, Denis Penman, Rich Morley and Yolande Sowerby. It has been our privilege to share our art with such an enthusiastic, committed and inspiring group of people.

Contents

Introduction

So...it's a Martial Art then?

In a crowded shopping centre, a predator sizes up his prey. Walking casually so as not to attract attention, he positions himself behind an elderly woman. The handbag will slide off her arm quite easily. He moves more quickly now. By the time anyone notices what has happened, he will be away into the crowd. Who will pay much attention to the ramblings of a confused old lady anyway?

The elderly lady is not confused but she is unaware of the young man moving swiftly towards her until she feels a tug on her bag. Without thinking, she turns and punches the young man in the abdomen. He crumples and falls to the ground. Winded and shocked, he manages to scramble to his feet as the old lady yells at him, attracting a crowd. Her bag is still on her arm as her assailant flees the scene. People nearby are congratulating her. An onlooker who saw the whole thing says she looked very relaxed throughout the incident. They ask her if she does Karate or something. She tells them she does Tai Chi.

~ ~ ~ ~ ~

Like most of the people whose real life encounters with villains on the street you will read about in these pages, this lady was a student of ours. At that time, she had only learned a short Tai Chi sequence or 'hand form'. She had never practiced push hands or the martial applications of her form with a partner. That week, in class, she had been learning a part of the sequence called 'step through, parry and punch'. This form alone had equipped her with the unconscious reflexes she needed to respond appropriately in an emergency.

Her story is not unusual. Although we have trained fighters who have won medals in competitions at international level, many of the students who have found themselves using their Tai Chi skills to defend themselves on the street had originally chosen to practice the art for its considerable health benefits and had not expressed an interest in the fighting aspects.

Yet, while there is no doubt that Tai Chi is an invaluable form of exercise for people of all ages, with benefits ranging from lowering blood pressure and relieving arthritis to improving balance and coordination and even increasing brain size, it was developed primarily for self-protection. It concerns us that this aspect is often submerged beneath its popular image as a gentle form of exercise.

We hear of teachers who tell their students that Tai Chi 'used to be a martial art' and others who insist that it was never a martial art in the first place. In some circles, those of us who teach a full martial syllabus are known as 'old school' or 'hard liners'. We have even been asked by prospective employers not to mention the word 'martial' in case it puts people off! Can you imagine any other martial art where this might be asked of an instructor?

Yet the seemingly gentle, meditative art of Tai Chi Chuan, or 'Supreme Ultimate Fist', was developed by fierce fighters at a time when the Chinese people were struggling for survival against hostile invaders.

We consider ourselves very fortunate that our own Tai Chi teachers, and their teachers before them, appreciated the importance of Tai Chi Chuan as a means of survival on the streets. One of them, Dr. Zhu

Guang, described Tai Chi as 'gruesome'. One of his own teachers, Professor Wang Zhizhong, in his book 'Taijiquan: The Tradition of the Thirteen Basic Forms', has described how growing up during one of these difficult periods in China contributed to his interest in martial arts and to his eventual position as an authority on Tai Chi Chuan at Qinghua University in Beijing.

As someone who has opened this book and read this far, we assume that you are not put off by the idea that Tai Chi is a martial art. You may be aware that it includes bare hand fighting skills and also trains practitioners in the use of various weapons, including sword, sabre and spear.

You may, already, practice push hands and martial applications of the hand forms or have an interest in doing so. You may be intrigued to learn how you can develop unarmed combat skills that make use of energy rather than brute force; internal power rather than muscular effort.

You may also want to know how your Tai Chi skills can contribute to your safety as you go about your daily life, or be intrigued to learn that even the simple postural requirements and mindful practice of Tai Chi sequences can heighten your awareness and make you a less favourable target for predators.

When these postural advantages and the automatic responses programmed by your Tai Chi hand forms are enriched by the practice of push hands and martial applications and an understanding of how the human mind works, your own and that of a potential assailant on the street, you can develop a set of skills that could, potentially, save your life.

Therefore, without apology, though with great respect for the thousands, possibly millions, of people worldwide who practice Tai Chi only for its undoubted benefits to their mental, physical and spiritual health and well-being, we offer you this book as a guide to the complete fighting system of Tai Chi Chuan.

Who this book is for

This book is for you if you are interested in how to use Tai Chi Chuan for self-protection and self-defence. It will be useful if:

- You want to know how something so relaxing and slow can be used for self-defence.

- You want to understand what's going on in class, especially what push hands is all about and how to take part in Tai Chi partner-work without feeling scared or silly.

- You want to gain a deeper understanding of the Tai Chi principles relating to push hands and martial applications of the hand forms.

- You want to learn how to protect yourself and others, if necessary, and how to avoid the need to fight at all, if possible.

- You want to know how to grapple someone twice your size or knock them out in less than three seconds.

Whatever brought you to these pages, we hope you find it interesting and of practical value.

What this book is about

In this book we will explore how Tai Chi can help you to develop the skills of self-protection and self-defence.

- *Self-protection* refers to all the skills, knowledge and strategies that can help you to avoid physical conflict.

- *Self-defence* skills are a last resort if none of those avoidance strategies worked!

Both are invaluable, depending on the situation, but avoidance is always preferable to conflict, if at all possible.

The main purpose of learning a martial art, in our opinion, should be to discover how to avoid a fight, while also being prepared to respond effectively if all else fails. This book covers much of the 'all else' as well as what to do if that fails to prevent physical contact. Physical self-defence should only ever be a last resort.

For this reason, our explorations will include a substantial section on how to stay alert and aware and how to avoid ever having to use your fighting skills in the first place. We will look at how to recognise some of the mind games people play, including the use of trance states to distract you.

If physical contact is unavoidable, then the skills you have learned through long years of training might improve your chances of survival.

The purpose of martial training is to install unconscious responses into your mind and body so that, like the lady in our example above, you can move without thinking. It may also help to acclimatise you to the stresses of physical contact, making you more able to deal with the 'adrenaline dump' that accompanies a conflict situation.

We will begin our seven step journey by looking at the basic skills, principles and science of Tai Chi combat and go on to discuss how you can test and hone your martial skills by practicing push hands and free fighting in the controlled setting of classes and competitions.

Drawing on our own experience of what could actually work in a real fight, rather than with a cooperative classmate or student, we will then look at how to use your Tai Chi skills to improve your chances of survival in an uncontrolled environment where there are no rules or health and safety guidelines and your only objective is to prevail against a concerted attempt by one or more people to do you harm.

If you are still reading, then that suggests to us that you are one of the few rare individuals who appreciate, or are at least curious to learn about, what is possibly one of the most effective self-defence systems in the world.

We trust that any new skills and confidence that you acquire from reading this book will not encourage you to take unnecessary risks. As with any martial art, no amount of knowledge and training can guarantee your survival in every situation but if it can increase the probability that you would prevail against an attacker, perhaps giving you vital seconds in which to get away, then your studies and long hours of practice will have been worth the effort.

If, better still, it allows you to avoid or control a potential conflict situation so that you never have to fight at all, then it will have been doubly worthwhile!

What this book is not

This is not an illustrated manual designed to train you in the specific postures and applications of one particular style. There are many of those out there already, along with videos galore, though none of them can ever be a substitute for actual practice with a range of partners, under the guidance of a competent teacher.

When we look at martial applications of individual movements from the hand forms or sequences of Tai Chi, we will be exploring principles common to all the different styles; our objective being to help you to think more deeply about how these techniques work, whatever style you practice.

This will not be a simple regurgitation of stuff you have read before, though we may back up what we say with what others have said and recommend these sources as further reading. Wherever possible, we will draw upon our own experiences and those of our students, and we will present our own ideas and understanding of what Tai Chi is all about.

Although we will explore the differences between force and energy, you may be relieved to hear that we will not be discussing 'mysterious energies', 'empty force' or knocking people over without touching them. Tai Chi doesn't need any of that in order to be awesome. It is based on simple laws of physics and bodily mechanics. When these are combined with an intelligent mind and patient practice, they become the ingredients of mastery.

Who we are

We are a married couple who have had the privilege of teaching Tai Chi for several decades to thousands of people.

We have also been incredibly fortunate to have studied with some great teachers, across several styles of Tai Chi, and we have had the added advantage of training and sharing ideas with each other.

Why we wrote this book

There are lots of books around that discuss the fighting aspects of Tai Chi but many of them are peppered with Chinese terms which can be off-putting or incomprehensible to anyone fairly new to the art. For some students, a kind of panic sets in at the idea of working with a partner, and this is worsened by being bombarded with whole load of unfamiliar words that everyone else seems to understand. Worse even than fear of getting injured is the fear of looking stupid!

Using all the jargon may make a teacher appear to be knowledgeable but it's of little use to the student if it turns Tai Chi into an impenetrable mystery that puts them off from the outset.

We want to share what we have learned about Tai Chi, over decades of study and practice, in order to keep our martial art alive for future generations. Our aim, therefore, is to set out in simple English, as far as possible, the most important things you need to know about how to use Tai Chi as a fighting art. We will only use Chinese words, such as 'dantien', 'jin' or 'jing' and 'peng', when we feel that this is unavoidable as there is no equivalent word in the English language, and we will explain in detail what these concepts mean.

We also wrote this book to help to demystify some of the less than helpful myths about Tai Chi that could lead to overconfidence in miraculous skills. This can be a problem with learning any martial art because it can encourage you to take unnecessary risks. The right time to find out that your favourite technique, that works so well on your friend in the training hall, doesn't work with a less co-operative opponent, is not at the point where the mugger's fist hits your face! We will at all times try to be honest about what is or is not practically useful to you.

How to use this book

Although it is possible to read this book through from cover to cover, with each section building on what went before, we have structured it in such a way that each section can also stand alone if you want to use it to look up a particular topic or skill, such as push hands or 'jin'.

For this reason, there may be occasional repetition of a concept to save you the effort of endlessly following up cross-references, though we have tried not to overdo this so that the mention of something you already know does not detract from your pleasure in reading the whole book but merely acts as reinforcement or further clarification.

The chapters, or steps, are presented in a logical order that allows you to check your foundations and explore the principles (Steps 1 and 2), gain a deeper understanding of the science behind them (Step 3) and how these can applied (Step 4) and then think about how to practice these skills in increasingly realistic settings (Step 5). We then take it out onto the street and consider how you might avoid conflict (Step 6) and what to do if you can't avoid physical contact (Step 7).

The principles discussed here can help you to improve your skills and understanding of Tai Chi but they will be of most benefit if you are

9

able to incorporate them into your regular Tai Chi practice. Many of these topics refer to skills and qualities which are felt and experienced as a result of many hours or years of training. There are no short cuts to Tai Chi mastery, and no book can be a substitute for actual lessons with a competent teacher, though we will do everything we can to help you on your journey.

What we think you know

In writing this book, we have assumed that you are already practicing an authentic style of Tai Chi with a good teacher. By 'authentic' we mean that it follows the recognised Tai Chi principles, as laid down in the Tai Chi Classics, and that it can be traced back to its roots in China, as opposed to being an exercise system made up by someone with no Tai Chi background who has just used the name 'Tai Chi' because it sounds nice and attracts students.

A good teacher is someone who understands the principles and can perform and use Tai Chi according to those principles.

If you don't have such a teacher and wish to find one, there are organisations that may be able to help. If you live in the UK, you can go to the website of The Tai Chi Union for Great Britain: http://www.taichiunion.com and have a look through the list of registered instructors in your area. Outside the UK you will need to ask your own country's governing body.

We are assuming that you will be familiar with the movements of a Tai Chi sequence, whatever style you are practicing, and that you are also aware of some of the most basic principles of Tai Chi movement, which we have explored extensively in our previous books, from beginner level in *Your Tai Chi Companion, Parts 1 and 2*, to an advanced level in *How to Move Towards Tai Chi Mastery: 7 Practical*

Steps to Improve Your Forms and Access Your Internal Power. This current volume allows us to go into more depth about the martial aspects of Tai Chi Chuan than we had space for in those books. If you have not read them first, or don't have access to them, don't worry because we will recap the main principles as we go along.

Step 1

Follow the Basic Tai Chi Principles

The martial skills of Tai Chi Chuan depend on an understanding of the Tai Chi Principles, as outlined in the Tai Chi Classics and other writings by the early teachers of the art.

If you have read our other books, or if you are confident that your Tai Chi skills are already at a high level, you might like to skim through this section as a brief revision of the basic essentials of Tai Chi and quickly go on to Step 2.

If you are less experienced and you don't have access to our other books at present, don't worry because in this chapter we will recap some of the main points you need to know, in enough detail to prepare you for the in-depth discussion of martial principles that will follow in Step 2.

The following are listed as 'basic' principles; basic not because they are easy but because they are the most absolutely vital foundations upon which all your other Tai Chi skills are based, so it's probably worth checking them out before we look at the martial principles. Patient practice of any of these skills, however obvious they may seem, pays off in the long run. Tai Chi skills accumulate slowly, over time, so jumping straight to the advanced stuff tends to lead to disappointment. As our teacher's teacher, Professor Wang Zhizhong, pointed out: "Haste does not lead to the goal."

So here, then, are the fundamental 'rules' of Tai Chi that you were probably taught in your first lesson and will have heard repeated at least a thousand times: suspend your Crown Point, sink and root.

How to Suspend the Crown Point

Of all the Tai Chi principles, suspending the Crown Point is probably the most important. There are two reasons for this:

1. If you don't suspend the Crown Point, nothing else works properly! It affects your ability to sink, root, use your waist and dantien and access your internal power. This is a result of simple body mechanics, which we'll have a closer look at in a moment.

2. Suspending the Crown Point is the one habit that's most likely to save your life by making you less likely to be attacked in the first place. The reason for this is that an upright, relaxed posture gives the impression that you are alert and able to handle yourself. We will discuss this in detail in the chapter on self-protection principles (Step 6).

So, since it's that important, let's be absolutely clear about what we mean by 'suspending the crown point'.

What is the Crown Point?

The Crown Point is the very top of your head. In yoga, it's called the crown chakra centre. In qigong or Chinese meridian theory, it's called the baihui point. If you want to locate it exactly, find the line that runs from your nose backwards over the top of your head. Then find the line that runs from the back of one ear, over the top of your head, to the back of the other ear. Where these two lines cross, that's the baihui or Crown Point.

Why do people get confused about the Crown Point?

A common cause of confusion for Tai Chi students is that there is another interpretation of the 'crown of the head'. This refers to the way the hair follicles are naturally aligned. The hair follicles on your head align themselves in a circular direction around a point that's usually an inch or two further back than the baihui point. For someone practising Tai Chi who thinks that the Crown Point is towards the back of the head, this misinterpretation can cause real problems with their posture because they are perpetually looking at the floor!.

Once you have found the actual Crown Point, what do you do with it? Well, firstly, aim it at the sky. Or better still, imagine that there's a piece of string attached to it and your whole body is dangling down from that point, like a puppet with only that one string. If you relax your legs and allow your weight to drop down towards the floor, as if the only thing holding you up is that imaginary piece of string, you will be suspending the Crown Point.

When people misinterpret the Crown Point as the point their hair follicles revolve around: they stand and move with the back of their head pointing upwards, so that their gaze is always down, about thirty degrees below horizontal, and they develop a kind of stoop. When a teacher asks them to lift their head, they then lift their chin while their neck still projects forwards and their shoulders are still stooped, like a turtle sticking its head out of its shell. Once they realise where the actual Crown Point is, and suspend that instead, they can relax down into a proper, upright stance and their postural problems dissolve away.

Of course, it can take a while to overcome old habits: you have to practice for a while if you really want to establish new ones, and the 'miracle cure' for unhelpful postural habits described above only works if your problem arose from not knowing where the Crown Point was. If your postural difficulties are due to other factors affecting the spine, such as arthritis, osteoporosis or an injury, then this might not help so much, though even people with a pronounced curvature of the spine have benefitted from suspending the Crown Point in their Tai Chi and many more have found that it can bring relief from back pain, particularly in the lumbar region.

Suspending the head in this way affects the alignment of the whole spine, providing you keep your knees 'soft' rather than locked out straight or deliberately bent.

Straightening the legs arches your back and compresses your vertebrae, making it difficult to turn at the waist, while deliberately bending your knees creates tension around your knee joints and in your back.

When your Crown Point is towards the sky, your knees are soft, your weight sunk down as if all your flesh is hanging from your skeleton like clothes from a clothes hanger, then the individual bones of your spine are free to move, the muscles around them can relax and you can easily rotate your waist and roll your dantien, two essential skills if you want to use Tai Chi as a martial art. We will be looking at these in Step 2.

Since some common types of back pain are caused by tense muscles around the spine, rather than from any kind of structural damage to the spine itself, you can see why, for many people, once they learn how to suspend the crown point properly, the practice of Tai Chi brings blissful relief.

With your head in the right place, you will be able to appreciate two other Tai Chi qualities: sinking and rooting.

How to Sink and Root

With the Crown Point suspended, you can sink your weight down. With your weight sunk down, you can develop a strong 'root' so that it is difficult for anyone to knock you over.

It doesn't work the other way around. No amount of visualising yourself to be a tree with roots plunging deep into the earth is going to help you to stay on your feet if your body is tense, your spine is out of alignment, and your head is all over the place!

The overall effect of being sunk and rooted is that you feel like a mountain that is wider at the base, or like a bear on its hind legs. It's an upright yet saggy, baggy feeling. In Tai Chi, it's known as 'sinking your chi'.

Where the mountain analogy falls down is that mountains are solid rock. They are immovable, which is useful if you don't want someone to knock you over, yet they are also stiff and hard, which is not at all helpful. Your solidity needs to be flexible so that you are able to move instead of getting stuck in one place. Even with your feet seemingly glued to the floor, your weight is able to shift from one leg to the other so that one foot is free to move. This doesn't mean throwing your hips from side to side, just feeling heavier in one leg than the other.

Training your 'other muscles'

A good position for practicing your sinking and rooting is the stationary qigong posture, or Zhang Zhuang (standing post), in which you stand with your feet shoulder-width apart, keep your body upright and your knees soft and let your weight settle down towards the ground. At the same time, you might raise your arms in front of you as if you are holding a large balloon against your chest. There are lots of potential benefits from holding this posture, not least of which is the development of your ward-off energy or 'peng jin', which we will have a lot to say about later. We mention it here so that you can notice something interesting; what happens to your muscles in this posture.

When people first try to stand with slightly bent knees and their arms in the hold-the-ball position, it is quite normal for lactic acid to build up in the muscles so that, after only a minute or two, their arms and thighs are feeling very uncomfortable. For most people, the natural reaction to this discomfort is to tense up and try harder to hold the position and resist the urge to give up. A couple more minutes and their limbs are burning. We have seen strong, fit men in reality TV shows reduced to quivering wrecks after five minutes of doing it this way.

The muscles that are causing this discomfort are the ones we use routinely and tend to rely on in our everyday lives. They may be strong but they tire quite quickly. When we consciously relax them, however, we don't simply collapse like a pile of jelly, we find that deeper muscle groups take over, and these are designed for endurance.

When we let go of any tension and allow our weight to sink down, we discover that we can trust these other muscles to hold us up. Better still, the burning sensation dissolves away and we may find that we can stand there for perhaps an hour or more without any discomfort at all.

There's a small chance, especially if you've done a lot of working out with weights in the past, that there may be a bit of trembling or shaking in the early days as your body gets used to the switch from one to the other but this soon passes as you learn to trust your deeper muscles and relax into your stances. Don't let any tremors put you off. It's not your 'chi' doing weird things, it's just your body adapting to something a bit new and the more you relax, the more quickly it passes.

In most activities, these deeper muscle groups are rarely trained but for those who do put them to good use, the benefits are enormous. Endurance athletes know all about them. Marathon runners don't keep going for over twenty-six miles by pushing themselves to sprint across superhuman distances; they relax the so-called 'fast twitch' fibres and let the 'slow twitch' fibres take over. Millions of years of evolution installed this feature in our hardware so that we could run miles in pursuit of dinner, swim across oceans and endure the process of childbirth.

These deep muscle groups are the ones we are training in Tai Chi; the ones that allow us to access our internal power.

Ideally, we can train and use both types of muscles to our advantage. Sprinting is decidedly the best option if you need to get away from some bloke with a knife!

Alertness

A consequence of the upright yet sunk and rooted posture is that it can actually make you feel more alert and confident; just as putting a smile on your face can make you feel happier. Feelings affect posture but it's worth remembering that posture can also affect feelings. This is why psychologists sometimes advise people to 'act as if'. If you're scared, act the way you think a brave person might act. If you are not very confident, act as if you are.

Having said that, don't allow your confidence to over-ride your natural instincts about potential danger and cause you to take unnecessary risks. That can be a problem with martial arts generally. As we will see in Step 6, the most important lesson martial artists can learn is how to avoid any trouble in the first place, therefore alertness is the most essential ingredient of self-protection.

Song

The Chinese word that describes being upright, with your Crown Point suspended, allowing you to sink and root and to feel alert and in control, is 'song', pronounced 'sung'. Because it is the foundation of all your Tai Chi skills, many Tai Chi teachers and authors use this word a lot. Since our objective is to keep this book jargon-free, we won't be using it again in this book but if you do come across it elsewhere, you'll know what it means. In the chapters that follow, we will assume that, when you practice your Tai Chi, you are in this state. If you have not quite mastered it yet, we suggest that you practice every day until it becomes your default setting!

How to Breathe

When we first begin to study Tai Chi, we can simply relax and allow ourselves to breathe normally as we learn where to put our arms and legs and remember the order of the movements. We can gradually begin to notice how the breath and the movements work together quite naturally, synchronising with the yielding and attacking, yin and yang. However, as we progress and become more confident in our movements, we can begin to explore the correct Tai Chi breathing, which allows us to develop and use our internal power.

The correct type of breathing in Tai Chi is what is often called Taoist breathing or reverse breathing. This has been dealt with extensively, with exercises for you to practice, in our advanced guide: *How to Move Towards Tai Chi Mastery: 7 Practical Steps to Improve your Forms and Access your Internal Power*

In case you don't have a copy of that book yet, or as revision if you have, here is a summary of the most important things you need to know about Tai Chi breathing. Please read this carefully as you are unlikely to find useful explanations elsewhere due to the fact that few people know about it and those who do often reserve this knowledge for their 'inner door' students!

Most importantly, you need to know that reverse breathing is NOT the exact opposite of abdominal breathing. Abdominal breathing involves allowing your whole abdomen to expand as you breathe in and then 'deflate' as you breathe out, which is very relaxing and great for meditation and other tranquil pursuits but it does not generate internal power for martial arts.

The opposite of abdominal breathing would be to pull in your abdomen as you breathe in and then push out your whole abdomen as you breathe out, which is as good a way as any of giving yourself an umbilical hernia! Potentially, it can also put a strain on your bladder and pelvic floor, with a possible risk of prolapse and continence issues.

Tai Chi breathing, therefore is quite different. As you breathe in, your chest stays down, your abdomen remains flat and the air inflates the lower lobes of your lungs so that your ribs expand sideways, your diaphragm moves downwards and displaces your abdominal organs backwards so that you feel a sense of expansion in your back.

As you exhale, you sink your weight into your legs and drop your tailbone, slightly squeezing your pelvic floor muscles and allowing your lower abdomen - below your navel (umbilicus) - to inflate. The upper part of your abdomen, between your navel and your ribs (midriff area), moves inwards as you engage the abdominal muscles in that area. The overall effect is that your lower abdomen feels like a football rolling down and under at the back and up and inwards at the front.

This effectively protects your navel and your pelvic floor (closing the 'chi gates' or bodily orifices in that region). It also has three distinct benefits for martial artists: Power, Protection and Precision.

Power

When you are adept in this type of breathing, your movements will naturally become more connected and powerful.

Protection

This type of breathing uses your abdominal muscles in a way that protects the area from incoming blows. It is therefore the basis of 'Iron Shirt Qigong' training.

Precision

This type of breathing allows better control of your hands and weapons, whether you are delivering a finger strike or controlling the tip of a sword.

We will return to this type of breathing in the next chapter when we discuss the use of the dantien.

Step 2

Explore the Tai Chi Martial Principles

Protect your Centre

There are two ways of thinking about your centre line:

The first is that some of the most important parts of your body are in a vertical line that runs from your forehead to your groin. On the way down, there is your face, your throat and neck (including your trachea or windpipe, your carotid artery and your jugular vein), your heart (which is generally central but normally leans a little to your left with its pumping chambers, or ventricles, directly behind your breast bone), your abdomen (including your pancreas and part of your liver) and your groin. These are all places that you really don't want anyone to hit you; so these are the areas you need to protect from incoming blows in a fight.

The other, less obvious, meaning of 'centre line' is your centre of gravity or centre of balance: the line through which an opponent can push you if he or she wants to knock you over. This is what you need to protect when you are pushing hands. It is also the line you look or feel for in an opponent if you want to unbalance them.

A skilful opponent will be looking for 'voids'; open spaces behind you or in front of you that you can be pushed or pulled into in order to unbalance you. In a shoulder-width forward stance with your right foot forward, which is the position that you are in at the start of most push hands bouts, your voids are the diagonals in front of you to your left and behind you to your right.

If you are pulled straight forwards, sideways to your right or diagonally to the front right corner, your front leg acts as a brake to stop you falling over. If you are pushed directly backwards, sideways to the left or toward the back left corner, your back leg is your brake. But if you are taken towards either of the other diagonals, you literally have not got a leg to stand on and you lose your balance.

Protecting your centre, then, doesn't just mean having your arms in front of you in a defensive guard position, it also means sinking low, shifting your weight and turning your waist so that your opponent does not get a clear shot through the middle of your body in the direction of your rear void; and it means not allowing your opponent any opportunity to pull you, by means of a pluck, roll back or arm drag, into your front void.

Use your Waist

You will know from practicing your forms that, in Tai Chi, the waist controls the direction of your movements. This concept has been explored in depth in *How to Move Towards Tai Chi Mastery*, in which we included lots of exercises for developing awareness and control of your waist, so in this section we will just summarise the main points that you need to know, in case you have not yet read that book or as revision if you have.

The reason people often get confused about the waist is that the word for waist is difficult to translate from the Chinese and is sometimes interpreted as the whole torso, so movements become stiff and robotic and people end up twisting the knees instead of turning from the waist.

If, on the other hand, it is only seen as the belt line, separating the upper and lower halves of the body, the shoulders and hips can end up turning in opposite directions.

So let's be very clear: the waist, in Tai Chi, refers to the section of your body from the line where a belt would go - between your hips and your ribs - to a line a few inches above that. It is what we might also refer to as the midriff region.

The muscles involved in turning the waist are the side abdominal muscles, which allow your torso to twist from side to side, and latissimus dorsi in the back. These are huge sheets of muscle that are much more powerful than the biceps in your arms. Therefore, if you want to throw someone sideways across a room, you need to use your waist rather than your arms alone, in exactly the same way that you would need to use your whole body to swing an axe if you wanted to fell a tree.

When the left side contracts and turns, the right side relaxes. When the left side has turned as far as it can, the right side takes over. The overall effect is like having a snake coiled around and through your body at midriff level, going in at the back and out at the front then surging around your ribs to form a figure of eight or an infinity loop, which is reflected in your movements.

The hips and shoulders naturally follow the waist and the arms trail behind like flags on a pole, with the fingers following last of all. There should be no independent movement of the hips or shoulders; they just get pulled along. When people don't understand this principle, they either move the whole torso stiffly, thereby twisting at the knees, or they become so unstable that their shoulders, hips and spine writhe, as if they are doing salsa!

The spine should, at all times, remain vertical and rotate, as it says in the Classics, 'like the axle of a wheel in motion'.

Use your Dantien.

This is one Chinese word that we make no apologies for using; it is so fundamental to everything we do in Tai Chi. The dantien (technically the lower dantien: there are three referred to in Traditional Chinese Medicine) is the centre of power in the body, even in purely mechanical terms, whether or not you believe in the concept of 'chi' or energy.

As a point, it is located inside your lower abdomen, about an inch (or a couple of centimetres) below your navel.

It is useful to imagine it as the centre of a sphere that fills your lower abdomen. Power in your movements is generated by rolling this ball, down and under at the back, outwards and upwards at the front and inwards under your ribs at midriff level.

Or you can imagine that your pelvis is a bowl half full of water which can slosh from back to front. If that description didn't help much, further clarification might be gained if we mention that certain reproductive activities make use of this motion!

This is why, if you see pictures of people doing Tai Chi with their back arched and their bottoms sticking out, you know that they are not using their dantien and they are not breathing properly, which means that they are not using internal power. However, this doesn't mean that you should strain to tuck your tail bone under you; just let yourself 'sit down' into your stances so that your tailbone naturally drops towards the floor, which lengthens your spine and allows you to 'roll the dantien'.

The breathing that accompanies this is the reverse breathing discussed briefly in Step 2 and is also discussed in more depth, with accompanying practice exercises, in *How to Move Towards Tai Chi Mastery*. The sound that naturally accompanies this type of breathing is 'hwa', though there are variations, depending on the direction in which you are releasing your energy.

Use the Square, the Circle and the Triangle

When you practice Tai Chi, the square and the circle are equally important.

The square is your structure. It gives stability to everything you do. If you want to build a Ferris wheel, you need to make sure that you have a big enough square or rectangular base and then anchor it firmly to the ground before you stick your wheel on top.

In your Tai Chi forms, you will already be aware of how important it is to have correct footwork, wide enough stances (so that you don't feel as though you are tottering along on a tightrope), a straight spine with the top of the head 'suspended' and the weight sunk down into your legs. This is the 'square in the circle'. Without this structure, there is no Tai Chi. When people focus exclusively on fluidity, right from the beginning, the whole thing tends to become as unstable as a jellyfish and has no internal power.

If, on the other hand, you go for structure in a big way but never progress to explore the circle, your forms will appear to be robotic: stopping and starting, one move at a time, with no fluidity from one to the next. This can happen if a 'square form' is taught first to beginners who then never progress to learn the circular version and go away with the idea that these robotic movements are all Tai Chi has to offer. They may even go along to other teachers and dismiss what they are doing as 'too flowery' because they are so used to their stop-start routine that they can't understand what is happening when they see the coiling and spiralling of practitioners who have understood both the square and the circle.

Tai Chi flows in circles very naturally and smoothly. This not only makes it a pleasurable experience and aesthetically pleasing as an art form, it is responsible for its effectiveness as a martial art. This will become clearer later when we look in depth at the various applications and their intrinsic qualities, but here are three examples:

The rim of the wheel

We use circles when we rotate the body in order to deflect an attack, in a fight or in push hands practice. The spine is the axis around which the wheel turns and the muscles of the waist turn the wheel. This is how we 'use four ounces to deflect a thousand pounds'. We will say more about this later when we go on to describe how to use a roll-back (in Step 4) and how to 'push hands' (Step 5).

The brick on a string and the brick in a sock

If you take hold of a brick and throw it in a straight line, it might travel the length of a room, but if you tie a piece of string around it and whiz it around your head a couple of times before letting it go, it will happily fly across the street. When you attempt to uproot an opponent, using a Tai Chi push for example, you would normally yield to their force, take it round in a circle and give it back to them; releasing it as a tangent from that circle. This is likely to be far more effective than trying to resist their force with brute strength and push back in a straight line from a standing start. From your opponent's point of view, the overall experience will be similar to falling into a cement mixer and being spat out again. We look at this in more detail in the section on momentum and inertia (in Step 3).

We can use White Crane Spreads Wings as a splitting action to divert an opponent's arms in different directions, or we can bring the upper hand around and inwards towards their temple, like a brick in a sock, providing that we keep the upper arm relaxed so that the downward pressure above your elbow is what causes the upward motion of your hand, like cracking a whip. Box Tiger's Ears (or Twin Dragons Search for Pearl) works in exactly the same way, using two loose fists to strike the opponent's ears or temples.

The dantien roll

Underlying all the skills of Tai Chi is an awareness of the dantien, around which all the breathing, power and movement is centred. This area can best be imagined as a ball which rests in the pelvis and can roll in any direction at will. Force can be issued as a tangent from the circle made by the rotating edge of the ball. The dantien can be described as the source of whole-body energy which is felt as a surge of internal power which can flow through your limbs like a tidal wave.

The triangle

A third concept to be aware of is the idea of a triangle or wedge shape which is created by your arms and body when you adopt the Tai Chi defensive guard posture of Lift Hands (Play Guitar, Strum the Lute/Pippa) or the close range, edge-on attacking posture of an elbow or shoulder strike.

In the Lift Hands guard position, the hands and forearms are raised in front of the body to form an isosceles triangle with a sharp point at the tip of the fingers of the leading hand and two sides that slope away and downwards along the forearms, allowing energy or force from an opponent's incoming attack to be absorbed downwards through the body or to be split and dispersed in two directions so that it can be neutralised and redirected.

Having spilt an incoming force at close range, the body can turn edge-on and deliver a wedge shaped attack with a shoulder or elbow like a spear head penetrating the opponent's defences.

Use Yin and Yang

The Tai Chi symbol, the black and white one that looks like two fishes in a circle, shows the interplay of Yin and Yang.

This concept is something that one of us learned from an experience with their teacher, many years ago. Here is her description of that event:

"I once asked my teacher, Master Zhu, if he could sum up, in just a few words, what Tai Chi was all about. Without saying a word, he just started to do brush knee and push as a stationary exercise, over and over again. I waited for a verbal answer but he just kept on doing brush knee and push! Thinking that maybe he had not heard me or had not understood the question, I asked again if he could explain what he thought was the essence of Tai Chi. Silently, he simply continued to flow through brush knee and push...withdraw...brush knee and push...on and on... while I stood there feeling a bit awkward and embarrassed, thinking that maybe he was deliberately ignoring me because my question had been so ridiculous.

"Then it hit me; the realization that will probably have you thinking: 'well Duh!' I asked if this movement itself was his answer. This time he nodded.

"Tai Chi, after all, is something that is experienced by doing rather than something that is learned from explanations, but it was more than that. I watched carefully as he flowed back and forth and finally asked: "Is it something to do with Yin and Yang?" He nodded again. "Exactly!"

"I had known about Yin and Yang for years. Other teachers had talked about it. I was even wearing a yin-yang symbol round my neck! I had thought I understood the concept: the business of never meeting force with force and all that. Patiently, he explained as he moved: "weight in back leg...weight in front leg; yielding...attacking; upward palm...downward palm; empty...full; breathing in...breathing out; yin...yang...not just in forms...in everything."

"On the bus journey home, I sat with these words of wisdom buzzing in my head. In everything! Yes I knew about the dark and light, male and female thing but everything?

"The more I played with this idea, the more I began to see it. How anything taken to its extreme leads naturally back to its opposite. If we exercise without stopping, we are eventually forced to rest. If we get too elated and excited, we eventually come crashing down. Inside an atom, electrons orbit the nucleus in pairs with opposite spin: if a subatomic particle appears in the void of space, it always has a partner with it which is its exact opposite. Matter and antimatter; creation and annihilation; life and death...everything!"

All of this from one movement: brush knee and push; the hand forming half of a yin-yang symbol in the air as it drops by the side, circles around by the ear, drops in front of the heart and then makes contact with the opponent's ribs and lifts him off the floor to send him hurtling across the room. Sometimes the most obvious things are the ones we take for granted and it is only when we look at them again with fresh eyes that we notice the profound truth within them.

Never meet force with force

Like two stags colliding and locking antlers, yang meeting yang is just one big headache; a stand-off at best until the strongest finally overcomes the weakest.

The rest of this book is really all about how not to do this. We will be looking at how to meet an incoming force in ways that allow the weak to overcome the strong; how to sense, follow, neutralise, and redirect a blow before releasing your own devastating response.

For now, the important point is to yield to an incoming attack. Meet hard with soft, yang with yin. This is not the same as being meek, submissive, delicate or fragile. Internally, you are strong, powerful and resilient; what the classics refer to as 'steel wrapped in cotton'.

The same is true of everyday life. The more you argue with some people, the more they dig their heels in. That doesn't mean that you should let them walk all over you; you remain strong internally as you listen to what they are saying, let them know that you have heard them, reassess the validity of your own argument in the light of the new information learned from their viewpoint, and then make your own point clearly in a way that they can understand. How many global conflicts might have been avoided with a bit of yin and yang, or give and take, leading to mutual understanding and tolerance?

For every high there is a low

In Tai Chi, the classics tell us to be aware of right when we go left, down when we go up, and it all sounds a bit confusing and mysterious, so let's think about what it means.

- If you wanted to hit someone under the chin with a see-saw, you would be unlikely to unscrew the see-saw from the floor and lift the whole thing up and hit them with it. It would just be so much easier to simply press down on one side so that the other side comes up with barely any effort at all, like a lever on a fulcrum.

- This same principle is used all the time in Tai Chi. If you want to lift an arm, you don't try to make the whole thing come up stiffly from your shoulder, you relax and create a heaviness in the upper arm which leads to a lightness that lifts the wrist. In our school we call this 'wearing the lead cape' but it all comes down to the 'sinking' described in Step 1.

- This downward pressure on the upper arms means that you naturally keep your shoulders level and your elbows low but, more than that, it adds vastly more power to your strikes.

- Always be aware of the opposites. When you move an opponent sideways, by applying a horizontal rollback for example, your power will be increased by allowing your waist to move in the opposite direction first and then loop back in the direction you wish your opponent to follow.

- The classics advise us to stand 'balanced like a scale' so that our weight can shift easily form one leg to the other. If weight is applied to one side of the body, the other can become lighter, enabling us to 'tilt' or 'wrap' the opponent while retaining our own upright posture and centre of balance.

- If an opponent goes high, you might follow and deflect upwards but then you are able to attack low as the groin and other targets are left exposed. If they go low, you follow and perhaps trap them downwards but may then attack high, for example with a back fist strike, followed (if your life depends on it) by a knockout blow to the jaw or neck.

- The concept of Yin and Yang also applies to strategies. If you are fighting a wrestler, knock them out before it goes to the floor. If you are fighting a boxer, grapple them to the ground.

The more you think about yin and yang in Tai Chi, the more you will come to understand its subtleties.

Look for Openings

Sometimes called 'doors and windows', these are opportunities to push or strike your opponent when they have momentarily left their centre line unprotected. If the whole length of their body is exposed, this is like an open door; if only a small area such as the chest is exposed, it is a window. One of the objectives in a push hands competition is to open up such opportunities by tricking your partner into leaving their centre line unguarded so that you can easily knock them over.

On the street it is more about getting a clear shot at the jaw line between the chin and the ear so that you can deliver a pre-emptive strike that knocks them out and gives you time to get away. Many violent confrontations are over in seconds.

Although we will have much to say about how to deliver pre-emptive punches and palm strikes effectively, it is worth considering that most of our elderly students who successfully fought off real-life villains - with the exception of the lady who did a rollback and flung her attacker across the street, another who kicked her assailant in the groin and the one who punched hers in the gut - did so by knocking them on their backsides with a Tai Chi push through an unprotected centre line!

However, in general, Tai Chi is more concerned with sensing, following and re-directing incoming forces than with standing your ground and waiting for your opponent to let their guard down.

Intercept with Arms Outstretched.

In a fight, guarding your head with your hands close to your face, as is often seen in western boxing, is all very well but if an opponent's fist gets past the guard, you get hit in the face, and sometimes when they hit your hands you actually end up hitting yourself in the face!

If you watch MMA fights closely, you may notice that the fighters with the longest guards often fare better than those with their hands closer in. A longer guard allows you to parry, to ward off, to drill and to intercept, all of which are Chinese Internal Martial Arts fighting principles that many people seem to have forgotten. This principle was discussed by Yang Ban Hou in his *Five Character Classic*, written in the nineteenth century.

Intercept and Strike Together

One of the differences between Tai Chi fighting and other martial arts is that it does not consist of a series of moves and counter-moves. Many fighters are trained to block an incoming attack and then go in with their own strike; leaving the possibility that, by the time their attack is launched, the opponent has already done something else.

In Tai Chi, you hit as you parry or ward off or drill so that the opponent has no opportunity to retaliate. Examples of this include fair ladies at shuttles, parry and punch, brush knee and push and needle at sea bottom. Yes, each of these is an intercept and counter but it all happens in one fluid movement so that your opponent has no time to reconsider their failed attack and come at you again. Also, as you will see in the section on 'jin' in the next chapter, there is a bit more to it than mere blocking and striking! We might better describe it as 'intercepting and issuing' via a whole slew of subtle ingredients, including sticking, sensing, interpreting, receiving, neutralizing and seizing, before we even get to the issuing bit, but to an opponent, it all happens at once!

Hand and Foot Arrive Together.

The weight transfers into the front leg as you strike. If the hand arrives first, the movement is weak because the power of the body does not accompany it. If the hand delays, the momentum of the body is lost and all you have left is the strength of the arm.

Whether the heel goes down first, as in Tai Chi, or the toe goes down first, as in western boxing, the principle remains the same: the weight transference accompanies the fist or palm.

These basic martial principles may sound quite obvious but they are very practical and are based on simple scientific laws. In the next Chapter, we will go on to look at these principles in greater depth, so that you can gain a clearer understanding of how to work with forces, how to recognise the difference between 'force' and 'energy', and what Chinese martial artists are describing when they talk about various types of 'jin' or 'jing'.

Step 3

Understand the Science of Tai Chi Chuan

As Grandmaster Chen Xiaowang has pointed out, Tai Chi is only a mystery if you don't understand the principles; when you do know the principles, and you can use them effectively, it is a science.

With apologies if you happen to be one of those people who hated Science at school, we really need to have a look at a few basic laws of physics that can help you to understand and master the skills of Tai Chi

Inertia

When an object is stationary, it takes a bit of effort to get it moving. (We all know that feeling). This is called a moment of inertia and scientists now believe that it is caused by resistance from a universal field of particles called Higg's bosons.

If you bring an arm back, ready to hit someone, and then try to launch your push, punch, strike or whatever, it's too slow because there's a momentary delay during which your opponent has time to do something to stop you. What's more, your attack will now probably be a linear movement from that standing start, which is quite weak in comparison to the way we move in Tai Chi.

To appreciate this, you need to know about momentum.

Momentum

Momentum is the tendency of an object to keep on going in the direction it's already going in, once it gets started, unless something gets in the way to stop it or slow it down. If you ever tried to jump from a moving bus and ended up with your nose on the ground, you'll have a good idea of what we mean by momentum! It's not that the bus dragged you behind it; it's just that you and the bus had the same momentum and you can't just suddenly stop by leaping away from the bus. This might sound obvious but some of us learned this the hard way!

As well as linear momentum, there is also a thing called angular momentum, which is the momentum of an object moving around a circle. As we said earlier, you can throw a ball in a straight line and it might go a few yards if you are lucky, but if you tie a piece of string round it, whizz it round your head a couple of times and then let go, it will go much further. If you have ever used a centrifuge, you will know how strong this force can be. Dog owners will be familiar with the curved plastic sticks they can buy to fling a ball for their pet, saving their arms from the effort and increasing considerably the distance the dog has to run. Shot putters and discus throwers also make maximum use of this principle, as do Tai Chi practitioners.

In Tai Chi, everything moves in circles and spirals. The Classics tell us to 'follow the circle to find the straight line'. A strike is more powerful when it is released as a tangent from a circle rather than in a straight line from a standing start.

Force and Energy

A crucial difference between Tai Chi and most other martial arts is that a Tai Chi practitioner knows the difference between force and energy and can use either or both, as required.

Tai Chi is an internal martial art, relying on internal power rather than muscular strength. Its principles underlie the other internal arts, such as Xing I and Ba Gua, in the same way that mathematics underlies all the other sciences, such as physics and chemistry. All of those principles boil down to one thing: the ability to use energy instead of force in certain situations.

So what's the difference between force and energy? According to Yang Jianhou, "Force is square; energy is round." But what does this mean?

Let's think about this like a physicist.

Force is what you get when an object is moving in a straight line. The more massive the object and the faster it is moving, the more force you get. This is why the external martial arts, including Western boxing, rely largely on muscular strength and speed. You generate force by tensing muscles in order to propel a limb towards your opponent as quickly as possible, although experienced boxers do relax when striking and may bob and weave to help generate momentum.

Energy, on the other hand, moves in waves. You generate a wave by relaxing your muscles and using your whole body to generate a ripple of motion through your opponent.

What effect, you may ask, might a shock wave have on the human body? We saw a perfect illustration of this in 2004 in a Channel 4 TV series: *Weapons That Made Britain*. In Episode 5, weapons expert Mike Loades carried out an experiment to find out how a poleaxe could kill someone on the battlefield at a time when body armour was so advanced that it could not be pierced. Even today, we use expressions such as "he dropped as if he'd been poleaxed"; but why was it so effective?

To find out, the armour was filled with a transparent ballistic gel of a similar density to the human body and then struck with a poleaxe. A slow-motion replay revealed a shock-wave passing through the gel, capable of causing concussion in the brain or damage to bones and organs in the chest and abdomen.

This is the kind of force that is generated through an opponent when Tai Chi is used correctly and it is why our teacher described Tai Chi as "gruesome". This is why some Tai Chi moves, such as 'drilling' and the 'one inch punch', should only ever be practiced on a punch bag and only used against a human being if your life depends on it.

To understand this difference between force and energy more clearly, you can try hitting a punch bag with your fist. The traditional way to do this in external martial arts, such as Western boxing, is to launch the punch from your shoulder with a tight fist, using power from your arm muscles and with the weight of your whole body behind it. That's a huge amount of force and it hits the punch bag in a straight line. As your fist hits the bag, your arm is tense and locked out and there is an impact with the surface of the bag, which moves it slightly and also sends a shock wave back up your arm and into your shoulder, though your muscles are braced against it. The amount of impact you generate depends on how big you are, how strong your muscles are, and how fast you are able to project that fist towards its target. (If you are into physics, you know that force equals mass times acceleration,

F=ma. If the sight of maths freaks you out, ignore the contents of these brackets and just focus on the previous sentence.)

Now consider what happens if you stand very close to the punch bag and place a fairly relaxed fist in contact with its surface. Keeping your whole body in the relaxed-yet-resilient Tai Chi state, breathe from your dantien and allow a sudden shock wave to be generated through every part of your body, focussed through your fairly loose arm and into the punch bag. What you will probably find is that, although there is no impact at all, since your fist had already made contact with the bag, the bag moves a considerable distance. Your arm remained relaxed throughout and was never locked out straight and there is no backwash of force into your shoulder, which was never involved in the first place other than as a link in the chain as the ripple surged through you and into the bag.

Now imagine that the punch bag was the abdomen of a person. If they were breathing properly, their abdominal muscles could easily withstand even a fast and heavy punch to the abdomen, but if your fist was already pressing against those muscles as you released your internal power, the shock wave would pass through their entire abdomen and into their back. If it was directed upwards as well as forwards, the shock wave would drive the air from their lungs in a similar manner to the Heimlich manoeuvre in First Aid. Potentially, it could also cause damage to the liver, pancreas, spleen, kidneys and heart.

We will look at Tai Chi punching again in the next chapter, along with palm strikes and other moves through which your energy can be released. For now, the important concept here is this difference between a hard, linear force and a soft yet incredibly powerful shock wave. With practice, over a period of time, you will 'get the Tai Chi skills into you'. In other words, the relaxed, resilient state will become your customary way of being and you will be able to generate shock waves in any direction, through any part of your body. We will say more about how to do this in the section on fa jin (or fa jing).

How long this process takes can depend on how much your body has been previously conditioned to tense up in a fight. In our culture, men especially are taught from childhood to be tough, grit their teeth, lift their shoulders and screw up their fists as hard as they can. You need to let go of all of this if you are ever going to get Tai Chi to work for you, and that requires a huge amount of trust as it goes against the grain of everything we are normally taught. Paradoxically, we only discover the evidence that it works by letting go to the point where we can do it ourselves. Cheng Man Ching called it 'investing in loss' and the pay-off is enormous if we really believe that it is possible and have a go.

We have, on many occasions, seen how difficult this can be in practice. If we take a group of experienced Tai Chi students who can perform relaxed, co-ordinated sequences, push hands drills and applications of all the movements of their forms and then ask them to do a little friendly sparring, we can pretty much guarantee that all of their Tai Chi skills will suddenly fly out of the window and we will find ourselves with a room full of tense people, with shoulders raised and fists clenched, firing jabs at each other like western boxers. It takes a huge amount of courage for them to override this primitive instinct and allow their bodies to relax to the point where their Tai Chi skills can come back online again and they can tap into their vast reserves of internal power rather than relying on hard resistance, brute strength or aggression.

And this is just in a class situation. It's even harder in a competition.

And that's just a competition! What would happen if they were out on the street and fighting off a mugger?

What we have found is that most of the students who have used Tai Chi to defend themselves on the street did not have time to think. They just responded in the moment using reflexes conditioned through their Tai Chi practice. It's the over-thinking that generates tension through fear or anger. Successful use of Tai Chi skills requires mastery of the mind as well as the body so that, even in extreme situations, we are able to use internal power rather than external strength: energy instead of force.

Jin

Although we set out to write this book in simple English and avoid getting bogged down in too much jargon and Chinese terminology, we have already explained three very important Chinese words: 'song', 'chi' and 'dantien'. Another thing we really can't avoid mentioning is the concept of 'jin' or 'jing'.

'Jin' is a very difficult word to translate from Chinese into English because it represents a complex concept for which there is no equivalent in the West. Most translators use the word 'energy', which itself is a complex concept and has a wide range of meanings from the capacity to perform work to the vitality to sustain mental and physical activity. It can exist in many forms such as heat, light, potential energy, kinetic energy or even, in the East, 'life force', 'prana' or 'chi', which complicates matters further still as, in Tai Chi, we often refer to 'chi energy', which is not what we are talking about when we are discussing 'jin'.

So, rather than cloud the issue by speaking of various 'energies', we will use the original Chinese word 'jins' in this section as we explore a wide range of the qualities, feelings and abilities they represent, drawing on our own experience wherever possible.

What is jin?

To anyone new to Tai Chi, the various types of 'jin' may appear to be mysterious or imaginary concepts that have been invented specifically to perplex and befuddle the aspiring martial arts student! All the talk about 'energies' appears to be vague and waffly and somehow unscientific.

However, the various types of jin are real physical processes that can be explained in scientific terms; we are just less familiar with them in the West than in China where, for centuries, martial artists have given a lot of thought to the forces or energy flows at work at every stage of engagement with an opponent and have given names to these.

Before we mention any of the Chinese words for these concepts, we will attempt to explain them as well as we can, using everyday English and a basic understanding of body mechanics and the laws of physics.

A circular strategy

The easiest way to understand some of the main types of jin, and why they are important to us in a fight, is to consider what happens when we make contact with an opponent in push hands. The 'circular strategy' we are going to describe here is more an order of doing things than an actual physical circle, though of course the physical movements of Tai Chi and push hands also work in circles and the process we will describe might often be carried out while moving physically in a circular manner, as in some fixed-step push hands exercises.

Let's start with an analogy. If you were in charge of a country and you suspected that the intentions of the nation next door were less than friendly, you could be forgiven for keeping your ear close to the ground and listening very carefully to what was going on across the border. It would not be a good idea to shoot off pre-emptive missiles in random directions, so while attempting to keep the peace by diplomatic means, you might also have the odd spy or two sending back information that could alert you to any hostile intentions.

Once your spies start to send home messages, someone back at base is going to have to keep track of that incoming information and get it to the people who can interpret it and decide whether or not it is a threat. If there is a threat and your neighbour prepares to launch an actual attack, you may need to neutralise or divert it and then launch a counter attack, using all the information you have available to aim your missiles at precise targets. Ideally, you might even use the other country's own weapons against them by turning them round and bouncing them right back, thus saving yourself unnecessary expense!

This is exactly the kind of thing that is happening in a push hands bout, and each stage of the process requires us to use different skills and abilities, from 'listening' to our opponent's intentions to neutralising his or her attack and releasing our counter-attack. In fact, we may even launch our attack on the basis of their intention, rather than waiting for them to actually make their move.

As soon as our hands or arms make contact with (intercept) those of the opponent, our whole body is 'listening', sensing and interpreting what we feel, alert to the slightest indication of their intention to move. To read your opponent's intentions, you need to be relaxed to the point where neither your own physical tensions nor your mental intentions, emotions or expectations get in the way.

We don't break the contact, we stick or adhere to them as if we were covered in glue and we follow their movements by becoming soft and yielding to any forces they may send our way, so that we can receive, neutralise and deflect their attack and then either lead it past us harmlessly, as in a roll-back, or give it back to them (issuing) in a way that does not allow them to escape. Ideally, we might lead them into a position in which they actually turn their back on us or find themselves off-balance, over-committed or generally unstable so that we can easily knock them over if we choose to. If we are really sneaky and unscrupulous we might even invite them in (enticing) and then slam the door in their face as they attempt to come through it by borrowing a little of their incoming force and using it to bounce them away like a rubber ball.

Every step of the process can be considered as a type of jin.

Types of Jin

All of these skills require practice until they become natural and instinctive. We have explored many types of jin and we have listed what we believe to be the most important ones below.

The Chinese names will vary, depending on whether you hear them from a Cantonese speaker or a Mandarin speaker and their spelling will depend on the type of translation method used (Wade-Giles or Pinyin). For example, just as some books will call the dantien the tan tien, 'duan jin' may also be written 'tuan jin', though they are both pronounced the same way. Don't allow any of that to confuse you, just find out what the technique or quality is and practice it until it becomes natural and instinctive, even if you can't remember what it was called in Chinese.

We'll start with the ones we spoke of in our analogy of the two countries at war, since these form the basis of the circular strategy in push hands (or sensing hands) practice.

Intercepting (Jie)

Adhering/Sticking (Zhan/Nian)

Listening (Ting)

Interpreting (Dong)

Following (Tzo)

Receiving (Zou)

Deflecting (Boh)

Neutralising (Hua)

Seizing (Na)

Issuing (Fa)

Enticing (Yin)

Borrowing (Jie)

(The word 'Jie' can be variously interpreted as borrowing or intercepting.)

If you think about it, you will see that what we are looking at here are processes which would need to follow on from each other in a particular order. If you don't intercept an opponent's limb and stick to it, you can't sense and interpret what they are about to do with it.

If you don't follow, receive and neutralise their incoming force, you have little chance of seizing and issuing (and any enticing or borrowing you might attempt on the way will more than likely provide your opponent with an even better opportunity to put you on the floor!)

Enticing and deception are ways in which you can encourage your partner to make the first move so that you can 'see what they've got' and work with their incoming force as they attempt to retaliate against your pretend move or take advantage of a fake opening, like walking into a baited trap.

When we launch our counter-attack, we can use various parts of our body to achieve the result of destabilising, uprooting and ultimately defeating our opponent. The eight most important skills in this respect (eight of the famous Thirteen Postures of Tai Chi) also involve types of jin:

Warding-off (Peng - pronounced 'pung')

Rolling-back (Lu)

Pressing (Ji)

Pushing (An)

Pulling / 'Plucking'   (Cai)

Splitting (Lie)

Shouldering (Zhou)

Elbowing (Kao)

Notice that these are being listed here as types of jin, not just as techniques or postures. 'Doing a ward off' could mean putting yourself into a good ward-off position in which your stance is stable and your arm is curved around in front of you as an effective barrier to protect your centre from an incoming attack, but that is still not the same as 'having peng jin', which means generating a feeling of inflation inside you that can lift and repel an assailant like an expanding balloon or surging tidal wave. This may be through the curved arm in front of you but it is also a quality that you can feel throughout your whole body.

These eight postures, techniques or jins will be described in detail in Step 4 when we go on to look at the applications of movements from the Tai Chi sequences or forms.

How you issue your counter-attack will depend on the situation and whether you chose to ward them off, push them over, press them away, hit them with a fist, palm, elbow or shoulder or pull them or roll them back, fling them away from you sideways or throw them onto the floor with a bit of 'downing energy'.

With practice, these movements tend to flow quite naturally from one to the other. For example, if someone is trying to push you, you might naturally roll them back to the side, which exposes their centre line and leaves them vulnerable to a shoulder or elbow strike.

If you do hit an opponent, you may do so more effectively by releasing your energy explosively (fa jin or fajin), which may be accompanied by vibrating your body, like a dog shaking off water.

With a good understanding of all the above types of jin and an ability to put them into practice, you could be an excellent Tai Chi practitioner, but our exploration does not end there. We will be going on to look at several other important applications and skills and the qualities expressed through them, some of which are also types of jin

Other types of jin

Raising (Ti) and sinking (Chen) are self-explanatory, as are opening (Kai) and closing (He). Some types of jin may already be familiar if you practice Tai Chi sword; such as Ti (uppercut or rising block) and Jie (in which you 'defang the snake' by intercepting the opponent's sword arm without making contact with their weapon). If you have practiced fa jin in your forms, particularly if you do Chen style, you will be familiar with Shaking (Dou) jin.

In your forms classes, you might have learned how to do a 'one inch punch' using inch jin (Cun) or 'cold jin' (Nung). If not, we will be explaining how to do that in detail later (Step 4).

Spiralling movements are essential qualities of Tai Chi, not least as a means of preventing an opponent from grabbing you or applying joint locks. You become as slippery as a snake. While spiralling to break free from their attempted grip, you can simultaneously drill forwards with a screwing motion to strike them with fingers or a fist. We therefore consider drilling (Zuan) to be an essential skill and we will look at it in more depth in the next chapter.

All of these types of jin underpin not only Tai Chi but also other Chinese internal martial arts and they apply whether or not you are using weapons.

The twisting (Cuo) power that comes from using the waist effectively is a fundamental Tai Chi quality and the art of Ba Gua takes this skill to the extreme, along with the spiralling and drilling motions described above.

Xing I practitioners may be familiar with Heng jin (crossing) and Pi jin (peeling). In Heng Chuan, the fist crosses the body horizontally and strikes from the side. Pi Chuan is usually described as chopping down with an open palm or sword. However, when you do a Pi Chuan palm strike, the striking hand first presses against the inside of your other wrist and then 'peels off' explosively with the force of a catapult, in a similar way to the child's trick of using a thumb and finger to flick a paper pellet across the classroom. Few people include this skill in their Pi Chuan these days, however.

You may discover references to many more types of jin out there, depending on the areas of interest of different scholars, practitioners and teachers. A great place to start is with Stuart Ohlson's book: *Tai Ji Jin*. You might also like to read Dr. Yang Jwing-Ming's guides to Advanced Tai Chi Chuan.

This current volume is not intended as a definitive guide to every conceivable type of jin and it is not for us to say which are the most important of those we have listed above. If your life was saved by doing something useful in a fight, it doesn't matter whether you used an obscure technique or something every beginner learns from day one, as long as it worked for you in that moment!

In what follows, we will focus on those skills and qualities that we, personally, have found to be essential and we hope to give you enough information to whet your appetite and allow you explore and develop further insights and interpretations of your own.

While all types of jin are important, three crucial abilities are warding (Peng), listening (Ting) and issuing (Fa).

Ting Jin

'Listening' in Tai Chi, is not just with the ears. Ting jin is the ability to use your whole body to sense the intentions of your opponent. Bruce Lee referred to it as being aware of the opponent's 'energy'; which does not mean looking for mystical auras, it means opening up your perception on every level, keeping your attention wide and being alert to everything that is happening with your opponent, especially through any point of physical contact with them.

For this to work properly, your hands and body need to be relaxed and sensitive. Tension blocks this ability (and also many of the other Tai Chi skills that require relaxed, whole-body connectedness). Tension is generated by emotions such as fear, anger and aggression. This is why mental mastery is just as important as, or even more important than, your repertoire of martial techniques.

Any real threat to you is likely to cause an adrenalin dump; a huge surge of stress hormones that can, potentially:

- *Give you extra strength.* You have probably heard of people lifting cars to save injured passengers.

- *Give you speed and athletic ability.* A lady we know, in her youth, ran several miles and jumped clean over a six foot high hedge to escape a man who was chasing her.

- *Make you freeze.* Generally speaking, no martial art is of any use to someone who is paralysed by fear, though as you will see later, even the freeze response can be useful in some circumstances.

Because of this primitive fight, flight or freeze response, remaining calm in a life-threatening situation, or even in a competition, may seem to be a tall order. You might not be able to completely eliminate stress hormones from your system at such times, but if you can at least step back from your thoughts and feelings and regain some control, it may be enough to allow your Tai Chi skills to function so that you can use the adrenalin rather than be rendered helpless by it.

Losing self-control in a blind rage is also very unhelpful if you want your Tai Chi skills to work in a crisis situation, though you may choose to act like a maniac if you need to.

Even if you are calm and relaxed, an overly-analytical brain can also sabotage your efforts to be sensitive! Trying, intellectually, to predict what your opponent is about to do is generally less helpful than sensing what they are actually doing.

If you have not already tried the one-finger sensitivity exercise in class, find a partner and take turns to lead each other around a room while only making contact fingertip to fingertip. You can try it with the person who is following having their eyes closed and then again with both partners having their eyes open.

Like thousands before you who have done this exercise, you are likely to find that it is easier to follow your partner when your eyes are closed and your brain is not interfering by trying to predict where he or she is going. Sight is our strongest, and therefore dominant, sense. Touch is an amazing sense if we trust it to do its thing, without interference. Our hearing also becomes more acute when our eyes are closed.

Your push hands skills are likely to improve if you practice, at least some of the time, with your eyes closed. Once you can sense your opponent's intentions in this way, you are then more likely to be able to follow, neutralise, redirect, issue or whatever else is appropriate in that situation.

Fa Jin

Fa jin, or issuing jin, is the explosive release of energy or internal power. The energy gathers at the dantien and is released outwards through the whole body but it can be focussed in whatever direction the mind intends.

Most Tai Chi movements, when you see them performed in an understated way, appear to be weak and ineffectual. This is not just because they are performed slowly and in a relaxed manner; it is because, other than in Chen style and some 'fast forms', the movements are normally performed without fa jin. However, although the internal power might not always be expressed, it is always available and implied: potential energy stored and ready for use at any time.

Professor Wang Zhizhong, one of the teachers of our own teacher, Dr. Zhu Guang, likened this storing of energy to the waters of a great river gathering in a reservoir. At any moment, you can choose either to retain this energy within you or to open the floodgates.

In Tai Chi forms, what appears to be the yang part of a movement, such as the push part of brush knee and push or the punch part of parry and punch, actually stops being yang and returns to yin at just the point where contact has been made with the opponent's body. This is the point where fa jin energy would be released if there was an actual opponent in front of you.

This is a very important point. You are already in touch with your opponent when you release your fa jin! To generate a shock wave through an opponent's body, you need to touch them. As you have seen earlier in this chapter, this is not the same as the external impact generated by a percussive strike.

So many people misunderstand this and attempt to put fa jin into their forms by simply speeding up the movement, tensing their muscles and trying to put more effort into the punch or strike. In other words, they are using force instead of energy and the harder they try, the worse it gets. If that's you, don't worry. We have all been there at some time. The solution is to 'invest in loss', as Cheng Man Ching called it. In other words, relax and trust the ability of your body to produce huge amounts of internal power without the need for muscular tension or effort.

Many years ago, one of us was trying so hard to find this mysterious internal power that she just kept on putting more and more effort into her attempts, to the obvious dismay of her teacher, who said that her progress was going rapidly backwards! Yet it was at this point that one of her greatest breakthroughs occurred. Here's how she described it:

"It was only after I had taken a week off to go away and have a baby and returned too tired to make any effort at all, that everything fell into place. Suddenly, I was breathing properly, I had understood what was happening at the dantien (dantien breathing is brilliant for speeding up the delivery of infants!), my forms were relaxed and fluid and I had access to vast reserves of internal power that I could control, withhold or release at will. It affected everything I did, from my Tai Chi forms to my calligraphy and painting. Suddenly, my

teacher was nodding with relief instead of shaking his head in despair!

"My forms were transformed too. Instead of trying to copy my teacher's movements and wrap my head around a million different aspects of what he was doing in his forms, I could imagine that I was him and move as he moved so that everything suddenly made sense, from the shape of the hands to the timing, the flow, the quality and 'feel' of the movements, the power and the energy. The Tai Chi classics that I had read over and over for many years were no longer mysterious but were something I could have written myself. I felt like the eagle on the wind, relaxed, alert and ready to swoop instantly. Mostly, I felt like the creature my teacher reminded me of: a panther prowling through the jungle; powerful yet completely at ease, every part of the body moving smoothly as a coordinated whole, yet able to explode into action in a second, should the need arise."

This is how fa jin feels. There is no need at all for tension. There is just a gathering and release of energy and an instant return to the relaxed state. Watch any video clip of a Tai Chi Grandmaster performing a punch and you will see how rapidly his or her body returns to the relaxed and ready state after the explosion of energy in the punch.

We are not suggesting that the only way to really 'get' the Tai Chi sense is to go out and have a baby! What we are recommending is that you surrender your physical muscular force in the way that you would have to if you were completely physically exhausted, because it is only then, when there is no muscular tension around to screw things up, that you can feel the stirrings of the whole-body power within you, which is seriously awesome!

A word about safety

Fa jin may be one of the most essential skills you will ever learn in Tai Chi, but do proceed with caution. That much explosive power being generated by your body can cause not only the shock waves you want to send through your opponent's body but also considerable shock waves through your own body that can potentially damage you as much as or more than them, if you are not doing it properly.

When you are using fa jin:

- You must be *breathing properly*, using your dantien, in order to protect your pelvic floor, umbilicus and internal organs. See 'How to Breathe' in Step 2 of this volume or the detailed exercises on dantien breathing in our companion volume: *How to Move Towards Tai Chi Mastery.*

- You need to *protect your brain* so that it doesn't shake about inside your skull like a pea in a tin and give you concussion. For this, your postures need to be stable and your weight sunk down, so that you issue the shock wave outwards and into your opponent, rather than upwards into your own head!

- You would be well advised to *open your mouth* so that you don't damage the delicate tissues of your throat and nasal passages.

- *Don't over-practice* your fa jin. Once you know you can do it, occasional practice is all you need. Even in your Chen style, you can perform your forms without issuing fa jin every time. You can keep the potential energy stored inside you and only release it when you choose to.

Peng Jin

Peng jin, or ward-off energy, is a feeling that permeates your whole body like a hose-pipe filling with water. Whatever metaphor we use to describe it, once you feel it for yourself in your own body, you will know what it is and the seeming paradox of attempting to be strong without stiffness and soft without limpness will become obvious to you. You will develop a kind of pliant resilience that is available at all times.

One of our instructors, a man past retirement age, recently fell down a stone staircase, across a small landing and down a second flight of stairs. On the way, he hit several steps, somersaulted above others and eventually landed on his feet and walked away without a bruise. People around him were astonished and asked how he had done it. He just shrugged his shoulders and said: 'I don't know. Maybe it's because I do Tai Chi.' No one was more amazed than he was.

Years ago, one of our own teachers was hit by a car while riding his bike. There was a huge dent in the car and his bike was a write-off but he walked away unscathed.

Now we don't for a minute claim that practicing your peng jin will make you invulnerable! These two men may simply have been lucky enough to have fallen in just the right way to have escaped injury, which might well have happened even if neither of them had been an experienced Tai Chi practitioner. On the other hand, it could be that their habitually relaxed-yet-resilient state helped them to go with the flow and bounce like a ball rather than stiffen up and break like a twig.

Peng jin, then, is available at all times, not just when you are performing a warding-off movement during your form or push-hands practice. Going back to the hose-pipe analogy, a stiff hose pipe with blockages and sharp corners is useless and may crack under pressure. An empty hose pipe, even a brand new, super-flexible one, is not much use to you unless you turn the tap on and let some water through. As Dong Huling said in his book *Methods of Applying Taiji Boxing* in 1956, when you are completely relaxed, you have no power at all, like a dead snake lying on the ground.

We need to wake up the snake so that it can coil and strike. We need a flexible hose pipe with the tap turned on. As the water pressure increases, the whole length of the pipe becomes strong yet pliant; filled with effortless, continuous power. According to Zhang Sanfeng (if our own recent translation of his famous treatise, via the German version in Professor Wang Zhizhong's book, is correct): "The most important thing is through."

The art of Tai Chi relies on your ability to animate your body in a fluid and continuous manner as if something vital and powerful is surging through your limbs. You can call this what you like but 'Qi' or 'Chi' is the word most often used. It implies not just a certain amount of muscular tone, nor even an ability to control your limbs in a coordinated way; it is more a feeling of storing, moving and directing energy throughout your body and expressing it through your limbs.

When you feel that your whole body is filled with this 'energy', you can choose to retain it or to release it. When you ward-off, you release this energy as an upward force that can lift an opponent off the floor in much the same way that a wave on the ocean lifts a boat, or you can bounce them away from you as if they just ran into a well-inflated balloon that you were holding in your arms.

The process of filling your body with peng jin, or moving from a totally relaxed, ineffectually floppy state to the state in which your body feels full of energy that can be stored or released at will, is what we, personally, refer to as 'priming'.

Your body needs to be in this primed state in order for all your other skills to work. Without peng jin, you will not be sensitive to the intentions of your opponent, you will not have the resilience to intercept, neutralise and redirect incoming forces and you will not be able to issue your fa jin in any direction, whether as a ward off, push or anything else.

With this in mind, we will now take a look at this process more closely.

Prime, Coil, Release

If you release a shock wave of energy through an opponent's body, it can be very sudden and it lasts for only a split second. This is much quicker than a traditional punch that uses muscular force and takes longer to reach its target.

In spite of its speed, however, your blast of energy doesn't just come out of nowhere. The potential energy (stored energy) inside you is released as kinetic energy (moving energy) into your opponent and this is a process that you can feel in your own body and also sense in others.

Here's an experiment for you to try:

Stand in a ward-off position but relax so much that your ward-off arm is loose, limp and as floppy as a punctured balloon. Now, very slowly, prepare to release your fa jin through that arm. Do you feel anything changing inside you before the release takes place?

Really take your time to feel what is going on inside your body from totally floppy to the final release of energy.

If you have a punch bag, practice your ward off against it but still take time to feel every subtle change that occurs before you cause the bag to move.

If you have a willing partner, ask them to place a hand, very lightly, on your arm. Again, very slowly, prepare to use your peng jin against their hand but stop short of actually allowing your arm to move. Ask them if they can feel any change in your arm.

What you might discover is that it is impossible for a completely flaccid arm to move suddenly and explosively. Something has to happen first. We call it priming. It's like a balloon inflating in your arm or water running into a hose pipe, giving it turgidity, just as a wilting plant stem is restored to life when you water it and its cells are refilled. A 'primed' arm feels quite different from a totally resting arm, and your partner may be able to feel this difference.

It is not the same as stiffness, however. Stiffen your arm and let your partner feel that hard tension for comparison. Then relax it completely and re-inflate it.

We could say that what you are doing here is allowing chi energy to flow into your arm. From a physiological and biochemical viewpoint, we could say that your brain is sending instructions to cells throughout your body to release stored energy from chemical bonds in molecules such as Creatine Phosphate and Adenosine Triphosphate, leading to increased muscle tone in readiness for the sudden burst of activity that is about to take place. Chi will do fine though. In Chinese terminology: the yi (mind), leads the chi (energy) which leads to li (muscular movement). It's the same thing, whatever you want to call it, and it always happens in that order. The chi goes where your intention leads it.

A primed ward-off arm is what we use in push hands. That's how it holds the structure without collapsing. But it's not just your arm that's primed while the rest of you takes the day off! Everything is primed! It's a bit of peng jin stored, yet not fully expressed, in your arm and also throughout your whole body. Most of the types of jin we discussed above, from sensing to issuing, rely on having some peng jin to start with.

When you are actually about to hit someone with your ward off, however, something else happens too. We call it coiling. As the opponent presses on your arm, it's like loading a bow or a spring or a catapult. There may be very little to see from the outside and the movements inside you may be so subtle that you had never noticed them until now, but they must be there in order for any external movement to take place.

It's like a wave surging through your body. It starts from your dantien, just that little rolling feeling in your lower abdomen as you breathe out, and it rises through you into your arms and also sinks down into the soles of your feet - as Isaac Newton said: 'For every action, there is an equal and opposite reaction' - which strengthens your root at the same time. If you go back to the floppy state, you can notice now that this is where the priming came from too.

So all it takes for that peng jin to lift the arm is for you to allow the wave to continue to surge without holding it back. You can do it slowly or explosively, it's up to you. Using it slowly, you can resist a huge incoming force or lift someone off the floor; using it explosively, you can send them flying across the room.

The point is that you felt it coming and, with a bit of practice perhaps, so did your partner. If you are lucky enough to have a partner who also does Tai Chi, the next step is for them to do the same exercise and for you to practice feeling their arm as they prime, coil and release.

Eventually, you may become so attuned to these changes that you can sense an opponent's intention to fa jin in the high speed setting of a competition and since you are already primed and coiling internally as you sense that intention, you can issue a counter force an instant before they release theirs. As it says in the Tai Chi Classics 'My opponent moves a little; I move first'. Of course, because you are already moving internally.

This is a very high level skill and takes lots of practice, but then so do most things that people are good at, from playing chess or football or the violin to swimming, juggling or performing brain surgery! That's what Gongfu or Kung Fu is all about. It's amazing how much natural talent people display after a thousand hours of patient, disciplined practice!

Now that you know what to look for and you have begun to feel this for yourself, there is nothing to stop you reaching that level.

Internal Power

'From familiarity with the movements, the ability to control the inner power gradually awakens. From mastery of the inner power, an even deeper understanding develops step by step. However, if you do not work diligently for a long period of time, you will not suddenly see the light.' - Wang Zongyue

Internal power means the ability to use every part of your body as one co-ordinated whole, rather than relying on the strength of the muscles of your arms and legs.

An arm used alone, while the rest of the body takes the day off, can cheerfully get on with the job of hammering a nail, but it would not be able to swing an axe without access to the vast reservoir of power in the rest of the body.

In Tai Chi, the classics tell us that movements are rooted in the feet, powered by the dantien, directed by the waist and expressed in the arms, hands and fingers. In other words, you need strong and stable stances, the ability to control your dantien, a flexible and upright spine, powerful side abdominal muscles and a relaxed and connected upper body that allows your internally-generated power to be expressed all the way out to your finger tips and even beyond into the weapon you carry or the opponent you are striking.

Internally, you can generate a phenomenal amount of power, and it is up to you how much of this you express or withhold, and the manner in which you express it. We are hoping that, by reading all of this book, you will be starting to experience your internal power for yourself.

If not, you may want to read our companion volume: *How to Move Towards Tai Chi Mastery*, and practice the exercises there. It is by doing these exercises and practicing your forms correctly for a long time that you gradually come to feel this quality of internal power.

Make the most of any opportunities to practice your Tai Chi forms and partner-work, in class or wherever you have space. Listen to any feedback your teacher can give you so that you can correct any errors that might be blocking your progress and then pay close attention to how it feels inside your own body as you make any necessary adjustments.

Even without much space, and without a teacher present, you can adopt a stationary position from the form, such as push or press. Settle into it and feel where the energy is coming from as you prepare to release it. If you feel stiff or the movement seems to be coming from your shoulder, start again and this time relax down until you feel it arising from deep within the core of your being. Feel it welling up inside your lower abdomen and surging out through your limbs.

You can express it outwards in different directions by using a splitting movement such as White Crane spreads wings, or Part Wild Horse's Mane', or focus it into a punch or into the tip of a finger, releasing it to whatever extent you choose, providing that you are breathing correctly and your whole body is relaxed and available.

As Professor Wang Zhizhong said in his book on the thirteen postures of Tai Chi, the storing of your internal power is like "a reservoir in which the water of a long river accumulates, powerful and stable, waiting for an opportunity to unload." When you apply your Tai Chi and release your power, it is "like an opening of the floodgates. Once discharged, the water flows over a thousand miles, sweeping away all the obstacles that stand in its way."

Don't just take our word for it. Feel for yourself this "relaxed and heavy force" as the great river surges through your limbs in your forms and applications. Keep practicing until all this stuff you are reading about becomes self-evident within your own body and you enter the "realm of freedom" – understanding and mastery!

Step 4

Practice Tai Chi Form Applications

In this chapter, we will take a close look at the general principles at work in a range of Tai Chi movements. We have assumed that you will have learned these movements as part of at least one Tai Chi sequence, whatever style you practice, and that you will have opportunities to explore the applications with a partner in class, under the supervision of your teacher.

Our intention is not to question what you have already learned from your teacher or to favour any particular style or method, just to allow you an opportunity to think deeply about each movement, including the structures, energies and dynamics involved.

You may already be performing and using these movements perfectly and everything we say may just seem to be common sense and repetition of stuff that you already knew. If so, that's fine; it just allows you to consolidate your learning in a structured way. If you find yourself disagreeing with us and you have found a different way that works better for you, that's fine too.

We can only share what works for us, based on decades of study and practice and our current understanding of the Tai Chi principles and the laws of Physics. We hope that you will read this chapter, like the rest of this book, with an open mind and if you gain any interesting insights that help you to use your Tai Chi more effectively, we will have achieved one of our objectives in writing this book.

The following moves are not gender-specific but it is worth mentioning that some may be of more value to a woman than a man and vice versa. This just comes down to basic anatomical differences and the fact that men and women tend to be attacked in different ways. In many martial arts classes, a common phrase is: "A fist comes in and you do this..." In a pub brawl between two men, that might be a fairly realistic scenario, but a woman may be more likely to find herself grabbed by the hair or neck or pinned against a wall.

There are gender-specific differences between the ways in which people choose to attack others, and these in turn will vary depending on whether they are fighting someone of the same or a different gender. The relative size of each person will also affect the type of attack they can use effectively. There are no rules on the street, however, and you just have to deal with whatever presents itself. Punching may be involved but you are equally likely to encounter someone who is trying to scratch, bite, grab, kick or slap you.

It is important to remember that these techniques are not used in isolation; they usually transform into something else. After rolling back an incoming punch, we don't just stop and wait for our opponent to make their next move. Unless our roll back sent them reeling across the street, like the mugger who attempted to rob another of our elderly students while she was on holiday, we may need to follow through by sticking to them and pushing them over, or striking them on the head.

Or, as two more of our students, a retired couple, did with a guy who broke into their house one night, we might choose to grapple them to the ground and sit on them until the police arrive!

This strategy worked well for another student of ours who found himself performing a citizen's arrest in order to prevent a very drunk man from driving off in a car. The technique he used to take the man to the ground was a double head hook, placing both hands behind the man's head and pulling him on to the floor.

Perhaps the prize for the most astonishing example of a Tai Chi student using self-defence in real life should go to the elderly lady who was passing a shop and saw through the window that two large and intimidating men were attacking her dressmaker. She immediately went into the shop to give assistance, taking one man in a head lock and then grappling him on the ground and holding him there until the police arrived. Fortunately, the other man ran away.

Though a fair amount of luck may have been involved in some of these cases, it would appear that sitting on people or pinning them to the floor is not without its merits as a means of restraining villains until help arrives!

Having said that, in most situations, one of your main objectives is to stay on your feet! Do not let the fight go to the ground if you can possibly avoid it. Your Tai Chi form applications are not particularly useful down there! However, Tai Chi principles can still be valuable in ground fighting situations.

Although Tai Chi does not normally include ground fighting, we would encourage younger and fitter practitioners of the art to explore these areas as well as their practice of forms and push hands.

Older practitioners may not want to sign up for a ground fighting class but we would recommend practicing lying down, rolling from side to side and getting up from the floor on a regular basis if at all possible, if you are not suffering from a medical condition that makes this impossible or inadvisable. This not only prepares you for self-defence but can also help you to maintain your general fitness and mobility.

In our experience, in mixed-martial arts combat situations, Tai Chi people do seem to have an advantage in being able to stay on their feet longer than practitioners of other martial arts, since Tai Chi is all about sinking and rooting and balance. If you ever do find yourself on the floor, however, stay on your back and kick upwards at your attacker until you have a chance to get to your feet and run away.

Each application of the Tai Chi moves discussed in this section will depend on the circumstances, the style you practice and the range you are working at, as well as your individual understanding of the art. Some styles work well at long to medium ranges, while others work brilliantly at short range or grappling range. Tai Chi generally allows you to get in closer to an opponent than many other martial artists are comfortable with, which can make their normal long range punches and kicks ineffective, though do beware of head butts, knees and body locks (bear hugs) if you are right up against them.

We will come back to the subject of which techniques work best at different ranges in the chapter on Push Hands (Step 5), but first we need to look more closely at the techniques available.

On the street you would not have time to think about which range to 'work at'. We hope that you will practice the following techniques at different ranges until they become natural reflexes that would allow you to respond effectively, whatever the circumstances. Our greatest hope is that you never find yourself in such an unpleasant situation in the first place.

The Thirteen Postures

We will begin with the famous Thirteen Postures of Tai Chi Chuan, which are the moves and directions of awareness common to all Tai Chi styles and sequences. "Keep the thirteen postures close", as it says in the song. Or as Chang San Feng tells us in his famous Treatise: "Practice Ward-off, roll-back, press, push, pluck, split, elbow strike and shoulder press".

We are also urged to consider all directions, in front and behind, to either side and to all diagonals, above, below and to the centre. This means being free to move in any direction and being aware of an opponent's force coming at you from any angle so that you can respond accordingly. It also means maintaining a wide sphere of awareness so that you are not so mesmerized by the person in front of you that you miss the one coming at you from behind.

Each move has its own direction, ward off being an upward surge of internal power while press is horizontally forwards. Fair ladies at shuttles can be applied forwards or diagonally and push can either lift someone off the floor or hammer them into the ground. Roll back and pluck may take an opponent towards you sideways and down but may also be used like a lever to lift a person by the arm, while a shoulder press or elbow strike can be applied in almost any direction, depending on the circumstances. Movements such as Part the Wild Horse's Mane can use a combination of forces including ward off, split and shoulder press.

When practicing each of the following applications, we recommend that you begin by practicing slowly and carefully with a cooperative partner and then gradually increase the speed as you become more skilled until you are able to use them successfully with an uncooperative partner.

Ward-off

'Warding off' means opening up some space in front of you with one or both arms forming a circle in front of your heart, as if you were making your way through a crowd. In a fight, it forms a barrier that can protect your face and chest from an opponent's incoming blows. In push hands, it bounces or deflects incoming pushes. When you are very close to an opponent, you can use it to uproot and unbalance them

It has a springy, bouncy resilience known as 'peng jin' (pronounced 'pung jin') or 'ward-off energy' and it is directed forwards and upwards, so that you lift the opponent's body or limbs.

It comes from the dantien, not from the arms or shoulders. Your shoulders and upper arms stay down as your wrists and forearms rise. It feels like a balloon expanding in your arms or a boat rising on a wave. The cultivation of peng jin is one of the key goals of high level Tai Chi training and it is present in a wide range of movements, not just in ward-off.

Although a good ward-off, with your weight in your front leg, can resist or bounce away a large force coming straight at you, once you have used it to intercept a blow it is usually best to yield a little into the back leg and turn your waist so the assailant 'flies off the rim of the wheel', as we will discuss more fully in the chapter on pushing hands (Step 5).

Roll Back

There are various types of roll back, depending on what style and sequence of Tai Chi you are practicing, what range you are working at - the distance between yourself and your opponent, real or imaginary - and the manner in which an opponent is attacking you.

In the Yang Style Long Form, for example, there is a considerable distance between yourself and the attacker, while the Cheng Man

Ching form is designed to train fighting skills at very close range or grappling range.

A roll back is literally about 'rolling with the punches'; not rolling all over the floor, which is the last place you want to be in a fight, but rolling an attacker off to the side as if they had run into a ball or cylinder that is spinning on its vertical axis.

At the same time, you move backwards, either by transferring weight from your front leg to your back leg or by actually stepping backwards, and you drop your weight downwards.

As an opponent's fist comes towards you, it may be heading towards your face in a straight line at high speed. If you just try to grab at the arm, you are likely to be unsuccessful and get hit anyway. The best way to intercept it is to ward it off with your forearm and stick to your opponent's arm (or cause them to stick to yours). Once contact is made, you can then turn your hand over to grip the opponent's wrist while your other hand or forearm puts pressure on their upper arm, just above their elbow, in order to prevent them from hitting you with an elbow strike.

At long range, you control the elbow with your hand, while at short range, you control it with your forearm.

Once you have your opponent's wrist in your grip and their elbow controlled, three things happen.

- *First:* you transfer your weight into your back leg (or step back if you need to and you are not doing fixed step pushing hands).

- *Second:* you sink your weight downwards, dropping your arms like rocks under gravity. When chimps fight, they often use their arms as dead weights to beat an opponent on the ground. Bones are heavy and gravity is strong on this particular planet, so do make use of it.

- *Third:* your waist turns, spinning your attacker off the rim of a wheel. In this way, we are using yin against yang, yielding to an incoming force but in such a way that an attacker is led into an empty space somewhere to the side and behind you. What you do then is up to you.

You can hit them on the back of the head, fling them across the room or onto the ground in the direction they are going in, or use press or push to throw them off in a direction at right angles to it.

Notice that you are not using muscular strength to drag your opponent diagonally into the void. You are combining three directions of movement (backwards, downwards and sideways around the spinning wheel) to create what mathematicians call a 'resultant vector' so that you can make them fall flat on their face alongside you or send them reeling away from you, with barely any effort at all on your part.

You are very relaxed, upright and balanced at all stages of this process and you are still protecting your centre line. In this way you are able to use four ounces to deflect a thousand pounds, as it says in the Tai Chi Classics. If a rock hits a spinning ball, the ball doesn't care: it just keeps turning and whizzes it away, without any effort at all!

Tai Chi makes good use of the laws of physics. It takes very little strength to perform an effective roll back. A lot depends on the timing.

The order of application of your three yielding directions is normally back, down and then turn, though these happen very quickly in succession so the whole thing is really one fluid movement.

A variation in our style is to sit back and turn and then drop the arms down in order to traumatise the opponent's elbow, though obviously this would only be used in the direst of emergencies and not in a competition or training situation.

Here are a couple of extra tips for pulling off an effective roll back.

- When you take hold of the opponent's arm, form a pincer grip with your middle finger and thumb. This is much harder to break free from than using all your fingers together. Try it and see for yourself. (Just don't leave your little finger sticking out.)

- In a close-range roll back, turn your palms inward towards your body as you go, as if you were wringing water out of two sponges. This gives you more control and allows you to roll the bone of your forearm into the upper arm of your opponent. In a real fight, this can be applied to the space just above the elbow or 'funny bone' where it presses on a nerve and can temporarily 'deaden' the arm so that they are less likely to be able to turn around and hit you with it.

As with any of these applications, you need to be quick and you have to be aware that the arm you are controlling is not the only weapon in your opponent's arsenal. Whether or not they are able to anticipate and prevent what you are doing - and how they respond when you do it - will depend on their previous training and experience.

You have some advantage in that their other arm is furthest away from you. If they punch with their right fist, you ward off with your right hand and roll them back to your right, so it is difficult for their left hand to reach you.

However, they also have legs and they may do something you were not expecting, such as run forwards past you and twist their arm in a drilling action to disengage your grip then whip your arm up your back, or barge into you broadside with a shoulder press followed by an elbow in your ribs as you let go. Or they could apply a press to knock you off your feet. Of course, you can do the same if anyone tries to do a roll back on you!

When you are training, do sometimes practice with an uncooperative partner and try to work out what you would do in each of the above situations.

A good exercise to train appropriate responses is the Da Lu routine in which you attempt to strike your partner in the face, they ward it off and roll you back and you barge into them diagonally with a shoulder press. Their response is to let go of your wrist and hit you in the face, so you ward them off, step back and do a roll back and they come at you with their shoulder...and so it continues. You can vary the type of roll back used, depending on the range, and you can add an elbow strike after the shoulder press if you wish. Real fights are not that simple but such exercises do help to train useful unconscious responses.

Press

The Tai Chi Classics advise us to 'be like an accordion, folding and unfolding'. Nowhere is this more apparent than in a Tai Chi press. When you master this skill, you become as resilient as a rubber ball and you are able to bounce people away from you horizontally with minimum effort.

The press is an extremely useful option if someone has you backed against a wall so that their body is too close for you to punch, kick or even use a knee effectively. If you can get your hands in front of your chest and one foot a little bit forward, you can use your thigh muscles to transfer your weight into your front leg and begin to lift your opponent's weight by expanding energy (peng jin) into your arms. As the assailant starts to feel as if a tidal wave is rising up against them, your arms suddenly explode forwards and send them reeling backwards.

Listening to feedback from our students over the years, the kinds of situations where this has proved useful have included care workers defending themselves against clients with 'challenging behaviour' and ladies fighting off the attentions of 'over-amorous admirers' at parties. How much energy you put into the press would depend on the seriousness of the situation. You might just need to open up a little space between yourself and an aggressive old lady, or a young lad who's messing about after a couple of drinks, but if there is any risk of serious assault from the person in front of you, you need to put them on their backside and get out of there!

When practicing this movement in class, problems arise when people try to use force instead of energy. We see people making a huge effort to press an opponent away by locking out their arms, stiffening their shoulders and leaning forwards. This is the opposite of what needs to happen in a Tai Chi press.

If you were to run into a large rubber ball placed against a wall, you would obviously find yourself hurtling backwards. The harder you run at it, the faster you find yourself sprawled on the floor at the other side of the room. The ball, on the other hand, made no effort at all. It just stood there while you did all the work. That's what a Tai Chi press is like.

Again, it all comes down to relaxation, structure, timing and the opening and closing of joints. One arm is in a similar position to ward-off, with your palm towards you at the level of your heart, while the other palm faces outwards and provides reinforcement to your hand and wrist. As the opponent's force comes in, your arms absorb it and seemingly collapse inwards towards your chest as your back straightens, your shoulder blades move towards each other and you breathe into your lower back. As you breathe out, your weight sinks down into your legs, allowing your tailbone to drop, your dantien to roll and your shoulder blades (scapulae) to move apart so that the area of your back just below your armpits expands like a concertina, sending a wave of energy through your arms and into your opponent.

Your shoulders stay down and relaxed throughout, and so do your elbows. For some students this can sound confusing; after all, we did say that your shoulder blades move apart and we are also saying that your shoulders stay down and level! The important distinction to make here is between your shoulder blades, which move outwards and sideways, and the tops of your shoulders, which should feel as if a heavy weight is pressing down on them at all times. You never hunch your shoulders and bring them up to touch your ears - just keep them relaxed and down and let your middle and lower back become rounded like a turtle shell as you release your press.

In any Tai Chi sequence, press is usually followed by a double-handed push, which is what to do if your opponent, recovering from being unbalanced by your press, decides to come back and continue the argument!

Push

This movement is deceptively powerful and, potentially, it can send an opponent twice your size staggering away from you. Out of the many students we have mentioned in this book, it is interesting to note that the majority used a Tai Chi push when defending themselves on the street.

A gentleman who saw off three aggressive double glazing salesman did so by pushing over the one who was poking a finger into his face. On another occasion, a young man who was attacked by a gang one night in a bus station used a Tai Chi push on the gang leader, allowing him to get himself and his girlfriend to safety. An older lady challenging a young man who had just robbed her house and was preparing to hit her over the head with a hammer used a push that sent him reeling down a hill in her garden.

A Tai Chi double-handed push has an energy called 'An', which is traditionally applied as a downwards force capable of sending a shock wave through your opponent and towards the ground. This can potentially destroy their root and send them bouncing away from you and it can also do serious damage to joints of the legs and lower back. For this reason, we do not recommend doing it in this way with a partner in class. Save it for the villain on the street.

You can either apply it as a push, by laying hands on your opponent before you release your energy, or as a double palm strike. Only pushes are allowed in competitions, however. Percussive palm strikes are banned because they are potentially lethal.

A modified way to do a double-handed push is to use it to lift your opponent off the floor and send them flying for a considerable distance. Again, this breaks their root but it does not cause them the compacting injuries of a downward push. Because it is directed upwards, it could be said to be using ward-off energy, but whichever type of push you use, you are absorbing an opponent's incoming force and redirecting it as a tangent off a circle.

As your opponent's force comes towards you, you don't resist it, you yield by transferring your weight into your back leg and lowering your arms to move in towards your chest and downwards towards your abdomen in a circular manner, as if you are sliding your hands around a large ball in front of you, inwards and downwards.

From your opponent's viewpoint, their attack met no resistance and it is as if they are falling forwards into a hole. At that point, you continue the circle so that, as you shift your weight into your front leg, your hands now move under the imaginary ball and up the other side, delivering a blast of energy into your opponent's body, just below their ribs and diagonally upwards so that you are, in effect, using their rib-cage to lift them off the floor.

Emitting your energy is like drawing a tangent off a circle. As your hands come round the ball, they can release energy as a downwards and forwards tangent, hammering the opponent into the ground, or as a forwards and upwards tangent, lifting them off the floor.

The circle your arms make as you yield to and then return the opponent's incoming force, can be whatever size you choose. You might draw them all the way in before throwing them away from you, or just a little and then 'slam the door in their face'.

Another, less well-known, technique is to push lighter with one hand and heavier with the other, which can also destabilise your opponent. This is sometimes referred to as 'The old man pushes the mountain'.

The same principles described above for a double-handed push also apply to a single-handed push where one hand is used to deflect an incoming blow or kick while the other is used to push them or to deliver a palm strike.

Split

The value of splitting techniques, such as White Crane Spreads Wings and Part Wild Horse's Mane, lies in their ability to confuse an opponent.

If someone has their hands on your neck and you just try to pull them away or prise them apart horizontally, you are unlikely to be successful if the opponent is stronger than you are. The human brain likes symmetry.

However, when we push one arm diagonally upwards and to the right while the other pushes downwards and to the left, there is a moment where the attacker's brain struggles to keep up with what is going on.

If you turn your waist at the same time, then this adds an extra dimension to the confusion and may give you an opportunity to escape. If you turn in the direction of your lower hand, your upper hand is now in close proximity to the assailant's face and might be able to deliver an effective strike to their jaw or neck and end their attack.

Your weight is in your back leg, so you can easily deliver a knee to the groin or a kick to the knee or shin or, better still, get out of there.

Technically, any movement where you are using two hands to apply pressure in different directions, such as when trapping an opponent's arm in play guitar, you are using a splitting action. The wedge shape of play guitar can also split an incoming force in two directions. When you issue forces in opposite directions round a circle, by turning your waist or by 'threading' your arms, your opponent may feel as if they have fallen into a whirlpool.

Pluck

Pluck is an odd word which attempts to describe the action of locking and pulling an arm. In that way it can be similar to a roll back but while a roll back involves intercepting an incoming force, turning the waist and deflecting the attack as if from the rim of a wheel; pluck is more linear and is applied by seizing an opponent's rigid arm and either dragging it downwards, upwards or to the side, or redirecting its force back at them.

When an opponent becomes rigid and their straight arm is trapped (arm bar) and under your control, you can either pull it (arm drag), or push it along its length, sending force directly into the opponent's shoulder. You can initiate a pluck at the moment you sense that the opponent has become rigid and take advantage of this.

Another thing you can do with an opponent's locked-out arm is to apply a downward pressure below their elbow while at the same time applying upward pressure above their elbow. This acts like a lever or see-saw that can unbalance them and even lift them up so that their feet leave the floor. This is surprisingly easy to do, since they have to 'go with it' to prevent a shoulder injury but, for this reason, you have to do it very carefully if you practice with a partner and stop when they tell you to or as soon as you sense that they are uncomfortable.

Shoulder press and shoulder strike

Like press, shoulder press is another movement which is extremely useful when you are being crowded by your opponent and you need to open up some space in order to kick or punch or elbow your attacker and escape. It is particularly helpful if you are smaller than the attacker. A taller person might go straight in with an elbow strike.

The idea is to turn sideways on to the attacker so that you can use your shoulder to push them away from you while your arms protect your centre line; one arm vertical with your hand protecting your groin, the other bent with your forearm across your heart so that your hand rests on the opposite upper arm. Your head turns with your body so that if your attacker decides to head butt you at this close range, it is the side of your head that receives the blow and not your face. If you time it well, there should be no opportunity for them to head butt you.

When you use shoulder press, don't lean forwards, which would invite your attacker to grab your head, pull it down and bring a knee up into your face. The idea is to remain vertical as you transfer the weight of your whole body from one leg to the other using your thigh muscles. Remember that your whole body is moving sideways into your opponent.

Once you have moved your opponent a few inches and opened up a bit of space, you may then be able to follow through with an elbow strike to the solar plexus and perhaps a back fist to the groin or face and then continue to beat them back by whatever means until you are able to escape.

In Yang Style forms, a shoulder press often comes after play guitar/lute/pippa and is followed by elbow strike and white crane spreads wings, a useful splitting and turning action to free you from an attackers attempts to grab you.

It is also worth noting that the same principle applies to part the wild horse's mane, which is a type of ward off that can also be used like a shoulder press before separating the arms to assist you in propelling the opponent away from you diagonally. The same could be said of diagonal flying.

Shoulder press reminds us that we can use any part of our body in a fight, not just our arms and legs, and we can launch our attack in any direction, including sideways. An important point is that we are not always hitting in a percussive manner with fists, palms, elbows, knees or feet; we are often releasing energy into an opponent and this can be released through any part of the body. When it comes from the entire torso, propelled initially by the thighs, it can be a very powerful way to unbalance an opponent.

Another very important use of the shoulder is the shoulder-strike or 'bump' in which the shoulder rotates forwards and inwards to hit the opponent during close-range grappling. These two movements are often confused and the terms shoulder press and shoulder strike are often used interchangeably but they are distinctly different techniques with different applications.

Elbow strike

The elbow is a useful weapon in a close range grappling situation. In a real fight, you can use it at any time and in any direction, depending on the circumstances.

When someone is so close up against you that you are unable to punch, kick or palm strike, if you can turn your body side-on and shoulder-press them, the transfer of weight into your front leg opens up a space so that you can bend your arm and jab your elbow into the assailant's abdomen or ribs, creating a further opportunity to follow through with a back fist to the groin or face, after which you might have opened up enough space for a knee to the groin or a punch to the jaw.

High elbow strikes to the head may be useful in some circumstances but raising an elbow that high leaves your armpit exposed and makes you vulnerable to your opponent's ward-off: they can simply step back out of range, parry and lift your arm and then knock you over. You are also leaving your centre unguarded, creating an open window for them to attack your body. We would only recommend this type of elbow strike to follow through after delivering a barrage of punches and palm strikes which have dazed them and caused them to bow their head and attempt to cover it with their hands. This sounds very brutal but you would only be using this strategy in a life or death struggle, not in a Tai Chi competition.

There are many different ways in which you can use an elbow effectively without leaving yourself vulnerable. You can strike with an elbow in almost any direction: forwards, sideways, backwards and downwards, as long as you are using the elbow appropriately and not randomly. You can also use the elbows for defence as well as attack. Do be aware that, although your elbows are extremely useful weapons on the street, elbow strikes are not allowed in Tai Chi competitions, though they are permitted in some martial arts such as Thai boxing.

Other Important Skills

Palm Strikes

Open palm strikes may not look very impressive to anyone without a martial arts background. This failure to impress may be the reason that they are rarely seen in choreographed fights in movies. However, they are potentially as devastating as a punch with a closed fist.

Punching someone very hard with a bare fist is likely to damage your own knuckles and render your hand useless for further fighting, while an open palm strike is safer for your hands but is still as effective as a punch from the point of view of an opponent.

Palm strikes are very effective when applied diagonally upwards, under the ribs or under the chin.

They can also be used to strike any other part of the body or head and in various directions. While slaps with a flat palm may sometimes be useful, you can also hit with the heel of the hand and outside edge of the palm, with the centre of the palm slightly concave. In this position, the hand can lift the opponent off the floor and throw them off balance. It can also be used as a percussive strike or when issuing fa jin.

Delivered as a pre-emptive strike, a palm strike to the jaw can potentially knock an attacker unconscious, as can a chop to the neck or throat with the outside edge of the hand.

Punches

The 'one inch punch' is no sideshow trick or manifestation of mysterious energy. It's really very simple; so simple that elderly ladies

85

in our beginners classes have been able to knock heavy floor-to-ceiling kick bags for considerable distances using this type of punch while traditional boxers whacking the same bags as hard as they can have barely moved them.

Again, it comes down to the difference between a linear, percussive punch and a shock wave.

When you hit with a fist, you normally pull your arm back and then launch your fist forwards in a straight line, relying on the impact to do the damage and potentially breaking your hand in the process.

With a Tai Chi punch, something very different happens. You can relax and place a loose fist against the punch bag, standing very close to it, and then sink your weight into your legs as you open up the joints in your back and roll your dantien, in the same way that you do with a Tai Chi press. Your joints open and close like a concertina, folding and unfolding, and your back, arms and legs are like bows; pliable and springy.

The bow analogy is quite useful as long as you remember that it's the opposite of what you might expect. A bow starts straight, bends as you draw the string and then snaps back to straightness as the arrow is released.

In a Tai Chi punch or press, the opposite happens: your back is straight to begin with, but as you breathe out and release the punch it suddenly sinks into the bow position, which is what generates the shock wave, and immediately straightens again afterwards. This bowed position is a bit like a turtle shell, with your tailbone tucked under and your shoulder blades moving apart, your arms and legs are already curved yet resilient and the energy from sinking and from the expansion of your back causes your hand to move forward by an inch or so.

And that's all that's needed because it all happens so quickly that a huge shockwave is generated, arising from your whole body, not just your arm. If your fist is against an attacker's abdomen when this happens, the shock wave goes right through their internal organs, which can rupture the spleen or cause damage to the pancreas or liver, just as the poleaxe did without denting a suit of armour. For this reason, we never do this in competitions or on other students in class, only into a punch bag.

At very close range, such as in a Cheng Man Ching style parry and punch, the direction of the punch is diagonally upwards from below the ribs, under the diaphragm, which 'winds' your opponent by forcing the air out of their lungs in the same way that the Heimlich manoeuvre does when you use first aid to save the life of someone who is choking. Such a blow could give you valuable seconds in which to follow through with a punch to the jaw to knock them out, or some other useful move to stop them coming after you. This works best if you are smaller than the attacker.

If you have used your left hand to parry a blow from their right fist, you may find the right side of the attacker's body exposed so that you can apply your right-handed punch under their ribs and into their liver.

For these punches, you need to be standing as close to your opponent as possible. If necessary, use a follow-step (as in Sun style Tai Chi, old Yang Style, Wu Hao and some Chen Style forms) to get in closer. At longer range, the arm whips out further but again the punch is generated from the dantien and not from the shoulder.

In either case, the energy is released into the opponent's body and then your own body returns to the relaxed yet 'primed' state, conserving your energy for whatever might follow. The timing of most movements, in Tai Chi is kind of:

...yin...yin...yin...yin...yin...YANG...yin...yin...yin...

Obviously there is a continual interplay between yin and yang going on and the energy will build and subside in rhythmic waves but the point is that, as soon as the energy has been discharged, the body relaxes.

As we have mentioned before, if you watch video footage of a master demonstrating a Tai Chi punch, you may notice that he is completely at ease until the moment his fist whips out like lightening with devastating power and then, an instant later, he is completely at ease again. This is quite different from what many fighters do: their arm locking out and staying locked out and tense for longer than is necessary.

Some of this comes down to experience. When people are new to the boxing circuit, they may be tense and anxious, their shoulders raised and all their force coming from their upper body. They tire quickly because they are trying so hard at all times to strike or to maintain their guard. When you compare this with an experienced fighter - someone like Jack Dempsey, Mohammed Ali or Floyd Mayweather - you see that they are relaxed most of the time, their punches come from their lower body rather than their shoulders and they conserve their energy until it is needed, then give everything they've got in that second when an opening presents itself. In this way, they are better able to 'go the distance' though, ironically, they are more likely to knock out an opponent early in the competition because their energy is so focussed and perfectly timed.

Drilling

Drilling is one of the actions which is rarely seen in Tai Chi forms as practiced in the West, but is very evident in Chen style, small frame Wu Hao style, Xing Yi and Bagua. It is a characteristic of the Tai Chi we learned from our teacher, Dr. Zhu Guang, who practiced Bagua and Xing Yi as well as Tai Chi, as did his teachers and theirs, going back to Liu Dekuan, who studied all three arts with some of the great masters.

If someone grabs you by the wrist, drilling allows you not only to wriggle free but also to deliver a strike to your opponent's face or neck at the same time.

It is a coiling action, your own arm circling the arm of your opponent as a snake might coil around the branch of a tree. As it coils, it surges powerfully forward and strikes like a snake spitting poison.

Drilling has the elastic, resilient quality of powerful Tai Chi. The arm is neither loose and floppy nor hard and stiff. It is relaxed and yet the fingers stretch towards the opponent. You might imagine projecting your chi from your dantien all the way out through your fingertips, like water through a pressure hose.

Although few people appear to practice this technique, it is a valuable skill, especially when delivering effective point strikes to pressure points in the opponent's neck.

In Tai Chi forms, drilling may be practiced in movements such as Repulse Monkeys, Grasp Sparrow's Tail and Fair Ladies at Shuttles. It can also be part of Wave Hands in Clouds, your hand drilling upwards to free your arm from a grip or to intercept a strike, and then turning over to grab the opponent's wrist and pull it downwards in a pincer-grip.

You can also use drilling in punches by twisting your arm as your fist reaches its target. This was considered to be so dangerous that, historically, it was not taught to beginners, only to experienced students. We trust that you will have sufficient respect for your partners, in training or in competitions, never to use this technique on anyone other than a real adversary who is bent on doing you harm.

Trapping

You may be able to trap an arm using play guitar/lute/pippa; with one hand inside your opponent's wrist and the other on the outside of their elbow. You can also do this using pluck in a similar manner to a roll back but locking the elbow joint so that the opponent's arm is straight and trapped between your two hands. In both cases, you can send a shock wave of energy up their straight arm and into their shoulder or pull them downwards towards the floor. In either case, you could then follow through with something else.

Trapping can also be used in a similar manner to wrapping (see below) which can trap the opponent's crossed arms against their body.

Tilting

We have spent most of this book extolling the virtues of an upright, stable posture in Tai Chi, yet now here we are talking about tilting.

By 'tilting', however, we mean unbalancing an opponent by tipping them sideways. This is something that is possible in a grappling situation when your arms are in contact with your opponent's arms. You don't lean sideways yourself, just lift one arm while lowering the other so that you rock your opponent off their central axis and destabilise their stance, allowing you to follow through with another move that takes them to the floor.

Wrapping

One interpretation of this is where you bring your arms inwards over the top of your opponent's arms in a one-two movement, and push them downwards, effectively wrapping them up so that your second hand controls both their arms while your first hand can come up the inside and hit them in the face with a back fist strike or a short, sharp punch.

This is not allowed in competitions except in full-contact fighting. In a real fight, while it would not be likely to knock out your attacker, it might buy you a moment or two in which to do something else, such as a punch or palm strike to the jaw or neck, that would stop them coming after you or slow them down enough for you to get away.

In a competition or a less serious fight, you might wrap them up and then apply a push to unbalance them or knock them over.

Another type of wrapping is to circle your arms in the same direction in a one-two motion (like a bowling action in cricket but without lifting the shoulders) so that your opponent is turned away from you with their arms crossed in front of them while you free your first hand and bring it round again to do a finger jab to the eyes, strike the jaw or neck or push against their upper arm or shoulder and knock them over sideways. We will discuss this further in Step 7, where we consider pre-emptive strikes.

A third interpretation is to wrap them in a bear-hug or body lock.

Guarding - The Fence

The main guard positions in Tai Chi are those in which one or both hands are raised in front of you in order to protect your centre line. In Yang Style, the best ones are Play Guitar and Ward Off.

The following relates to situations in which you find yourself face to face with an unarmed hostile person. Facing someone who is holding a knife or a gun is an entirely different matter!

Self-defence expert Geoff Thompson has spent years writing books and running courses in self-protection based on what he has learned over many years of practice. We strongly advise you to watch his video clips on YouTube, and also those of fellow expert Peter Consterdine, if you can, particularly those that show you how to use 'The Fence'.

Points to remember, from a Tai Chi viewpoint, are:

- Don't make your guard position too obvious. The idea is to control the space between yourself and your opponent without your opponent knowing the he or she is being controlled. If you start doing overtly martial-arts-style posturing, you will either make them laugh or make them more determined to control you. Be subtle.

- Keep your palms open in what would appear to onlookers to be a placatory gesture. Witnesses remember what they saw rather than what they heard. If you have fists up, they will think you started it, even if you are saying, "OK mate; let's not have any trouble."

- Stay relaxed and at ease yet primed so that you can instantly respond to any attempt to get past your guard.

- Don't let your guard down. If your hands fall to your sides, you are wide open and it takes too long to get them back up again. In less than a second, your opponent can cross the space and be in your face. Don't let it happen.

- Give your opponent an honourable way out, if you can. Geoff Thompson calls this 'loopholing'. People may not want a fight but don't want to lose face by backing down.

- If they try to come through your guard then, technically, they have made the first move and you are legally justified in using a pre-emptive strike to knock them out or disorientate them sufficiently so that you can either escape or follow through with other blows until you are able to escape.

- Don't hesitate and wait for them to actually hurt you. If there's even the slightest suspicion in your mind that they intend to do you harm, just strike them!

The law is on your side if you use 'reasonable force' to protect yourself from an assault. If you are attacked by a little old lady or a child in a temper tantrum, there are gentle ways to fend them off, but if your assailant is a serial killer, then ANYTHING you do to them in order to stay alive is 'reasonable force'.

While we recommend using a fence or guard, it is worth mentioning that skilled fighters may leave a space in their centre line in order to entice the attacker in. This is a trap in order to get them to commit to their attack. You might use this in competitions but in a real-life desperate situation you would have to be incredibly skilled, confident and possibly very lucky to pull this off effectively so if in doubt, use a guard.

We will discuss this subject in more detail in Step 7.

Kicking

Depending on style, Tai Chi kicks range from graceful head-high toe kicks and spinning displays of aerial acrobatics, to seemingly half-hearted efforts that barely clear the floor. As with many Tai Chi movements, the ability to impress is not necessarily an indication of usefulness in combat!

In a fight, with excellent timing, lots of luck and perhaps a few prayers for good measure, you might manage to take down an aggressive assailant with a flying kick to the head. More likely, you will find yourself flat on your back with your opponent on top of you.

Those apparently ineffectual toe kicks to the shin, however, can be very painful if delivered with a hard shoe and sufficient force. If your shoes are soft, the same thing can be achieved with the side of a foot or a heel. Better still, if you can reach it, go for the knee. If you take their knee out, they won't be coming after you in a hurry. Again, this applies only to life-or death struggles. In a competition, you are there to test your skills against a respected opponent, not to cause them serious injury.

Sweeping the kidneys with a lotus kick might look good on a video demo but it would not be our recommended option when it comes to practicality. (There are quite a few moves in this category, not least of which is any attempt to use a hand to strike an opponent in the foot, which is about as good as giving them your head to play with!)

If, on the other hand, your opponent tries a high kick on you, you might like to help it on its way in an upward direction so that they fall backwards onto the floor; or, since their foot is level with your neck, you might choose to walk forward with their leg above your shoulder and select from the range of useful targets available, not least of which is their groin!

If you ever spent some time sitting on the floor while someone held your foot in the air, you will appreciate the difficulty in making any type of comeback after an unsuccessful kick.

In general: Kicks: keep them low, keep them simple, and keep them fast!

Repulse Monkeys

While many people these days see this movement as a lovely meditative qigong exercise where you gather up a big ball of energy and roll it forwards over your other hand, repulse monkeys is one of the most devastating movements in the whole Tai Chi Chuan repertoire.

What you are doing is grabbing your attacker by the clothing at the front of their neck and pulling them towards you as you step backwards; effectively doubling the power of the open palm strike that you simultaneously deliver, forwards and upwards under their chin, forcing their head backwards, or hit them in the face, eyes, nose or throat.

It can also be used to step back, deflect a blow and grab the opponent's wrist or arm, while striking them with your other hand.

Interestingly, when you watch the way that practitioners of other martial arts 'mark' their opponent by reaching out one arm as if to judge the distance before striking with the other, it is clear that this may have originally been intended to grab the opponent and pull them in towards the fist, as in Repulse Monkeys.

Fair Ladies at Shuttles

Fair Ladies at Shuttles (or, as Google Translate would have it, Beautiful Weaver) is an extremely powerful movement, if you are quick enough to pull it off in a fight. Although it can be used in a linear manner towards your opponent, its real strength lies in its ability to get around the outside of your opponent and strike them from a vulnerable angle which they cannot defend.

You have to be quick and come straight back in at them from the diagonal so that they don't have an opportunity to see what you are doing and turn with you as you sidestep.

Fair Ladies is a good example of the Tai Chi principle of intercept and strike together (using a parry or ward off rather than a hard block). As one arm rises to intercept and deflect an attack, the other reaches the opponent's rib cage to deliver a palm strike or push to the ribs, or a drilling strike to the liver. The top hand can be used simply for deflection or it can roll and assist with a double-handed push or double palm strike by connecting with the opponent's face, jaw or shoulder.

However it is used, the movement is powered through the legs, dantien and waist, not just the arms, and the body is able to twist so that the force issued can hit the opponent from the diagonal, making it difficult to counter.

The amount of force generated by Fair Ladies at Shuttles is considerable and it can be issued in such a way as to catch the opponent at an awkward angle, leaving them vulnerable, off-balance and liable to stumble and fall. Even a small person can send a large opponent reeling across a room with this movement and therefore in a class situation, it should be used with care and never with full fa jin on a partner The drilling action should never be used except on a punch bag or in a real life-or-death struggle with an attacker, unless your training partner is wearing body armour. Even if your partner is wearing body armour, the shock wave generated by using your fa jin in this position could cause internal damage and the unbalancing could result in an ankle injury.

In a real fight, some of the above techniques could be useful and, for that reason, we recommend that you practice them until they become second nature. We also strongly recommend that you get used to working with various partners via regular practice of pushing hands (or sensing hands), which we will discuss in detail in the next chapter.

Step 5

Practice Push Hands (Sensing Hands)

If you are practicing Tai Chi, you may or may not have some experience of the partner exercise of 'pushing hands', 'push hands' or 'sensing hands'. Whichever term you use to describe it, it is neither all about pushing, which is contrary to the Tai Chi principles of yielding and listening, nor all about sensing, which makes it sound like a soft and relaxing partner exercise and neglects to mention the eventual counter-attack. Tai Chi is all about balance between extremes, therefore sensing what your partner is doing is as important as your response, if not more so.

Not all teachers include push hands practice in their classes, as most students are attracted to Tai Chi for health and relaxation. Some teachers have never practiced it themselves and therefore only ever teach forms.

This is unfortunate since it neglects an opportunity to explore the art more fully by putting forms into practice and gaining insights which deepen the appreciation of the forms. Tai Chi without physical contact with another person is the equivalent of trying to learn medicine without ever meeting a patient or learning to cook without tasting the food. Practicing sequences does form a substantial part of Tai Chi training, but without doing some work with a partner, you only have half an art.

Tai Chi, first and foremost, was developed for self-defence and combat and there are levels of training ranging from gentle sensitivity exercises to full contact fighting ('San Shou' or 'San Da'), which is the nearest equivalent, in controlled conditions, to an actual fight on the street.

Historically, applications of the forms would be practiced as realistically as possible, with classmates approaching from different directions so that the skills had to be applied for self-defence. Push Hands drills (Tui Shou) came later but are invaluable for slowing down contact with a cooperative and respectful partner, allowing time to think carefully about what you are sensing and feeling. In this way, both partners can learn some very useful lessons without the risk of injury.

Basic Soft Exercises

These include the finger-sensitivity exercise, which we mentioned in the section on Ting jin. You may have done it in class. It's the one where you close your eyes and your partner leads you around the room by just touching the tip of one finger.

There are also gentle 'following exercises' or 'sticking hands' in which you make contact with each other's hands and arms and gently follow each other's movements. This can naturally lead on to a slightly more demanding exercise, where you are still sticking but also alert to opportunities to get past each other's defences.

Another soft exercise is gentle body pushing. Your partner sinks and roots while you attempt to unbalance him or her by pushing on various parts of the body. In this way, you learn how to unbalance someone by finding their centre line and issuing gentle force in that direction. By allowing your partner to push you in this way, you learn how to keep your balance by sinking and rooting, and how to protect your centre line and deflect an incoming force by turning your waist.

These may seem to be weak and easy options compared with 'proper fighting' but they are not to be sneered at since they are essential preparation for what is to come.

When you can suspend the crown-point, relax, sink, root, turn your waist properly and do a decent ward off, you are ready to learn the art of push hands.

If you already practice push hands, you might still find the following section to be of interest, so do take a look at how it compares with what you are doing. We will largely focus on Yang Style push hands but we are aware of the variations used in Chen, Wu and other styles. While Chen push hands has very long, deep stances and partners are almost edge on to each other and Wu stylists tend to lean forwards towards each other more than the upright Yang and Chen stylists, many of the principles are the same, and it is from practicing these drills, routines and combative sports that you come to appreciate some of the higher level Tai Chi fighting principles that we discuss elsewhere in this book.

Single Fixed Step Push Hands

This is the simplest type of push hands, in which both partners face each other in a forward stance, one arm in ward-off position, and make contact with each other at the wrist. The other hand either stays at their side or behind their back as they attempt to unbalance each other with just one hand/arm, without moving their feet. Most competitions do not include this category but it is a valuable training exercise, as it is the foundation on which double hand fixed step and moving step skills are based. You could say that this is where Tai Chi fighters first cut their teeth and learn to walk.

Keep it soft and gentle, like play, to begin with. If you try too hard, or become overly concerned with your performance, you will tense up and miss some of the important lessons that can be learned.

The keys to mastery of this skill are:

- *Structure.* No surprises here, after everything that has already been said in this book and its companion volumes! However, this is the point at which all the structural points you have practiced in your forms become crucial to your ability to maintain your balance and push hands effectively with a variety of partners. Keep your feet shoulder-width apart in your forward stance, suspend your crown-point, sink, root and use your waist, rather than moving your arm independently.

- *Maintain your ward-off* so that you *protect your centre line* at all times. Beginners tend to struggle with this concept and will usually move their arm to one side, leaving their chest unguarded, instead of keeping their wrist in front of their sternum and using their waist to deflect the incoming force.

- '*Sit the wrist*'. Keep your hand relaxed and only offer your opponent the end of your arm bone to push on. A classic mistake that beginners make is that they tense up the hand and try to use it to drag their opponent around. All they succeed in doing is giving their opponent their stiff hand as something else to push on, allowing them to trap the arm and take it across the neck or body. This is something that is usually learned the hard way when you find yourself knocked over or pinned against a wall. You can save yourself this embarrassment by learning this point early and making it the default setting for your hand in push hands drills, bouts and competitions.

- *Timing* is important in push hands. It is all about playing with incoming forces. If your opponent doesn't move, then neither do you! You need their incoming force to work with. When they push on your arm, you yield and deflect and return with your response. Don't just attack them with force as they come at you or yield before they start to push. However, sometimes, if neither person is willing to make the first move, it may be necessary to do a small 'dummy push' just to get things moving and 'see what they've got'.

- *Use your waist* to deflect your partner's incoming push. When you turn, it should be to what seems to be the awkward side. For example, if your right leg is forward, you turn to the right, though this may seem counter-intuitive. If you turn the other way, you open up your body to a push straight through your centre line as they collapse your arm in against your chest or throat.

- *Use the three circles.* There are three structural circles that you need to be aware of from the moment you begin to practice push hands, all of them horizontal and on the same plane as your heart. The best way to imagine them is as viewed from above. The first is the circle your arm makes as you ward off, as if holding a balloon against your chest. The other two have your spine as their central axis: a large circle with its circumference touching the back of your wrist as you ward off, and a small circle whose circumference touches your breast bone. You can choose whether to ward off and rotate so that your opponent spins off the rim of the big circle, or you can bring your hand right in to touch your chest and spin them off the small circle. The space between the large and small circles is a no-go area, since trying to hold someone off with a bent (rather than curved) elbow means you suddenly find yourself having to use brute force instead of easy circular dynamics. A circle is a strong, resilient structure, whereas a bent arm can be collapsed very easily. However, with practice, you can shrink the diameter of the large circle by dropping your elbow rather than bending it, so that it feels like you have a balloon in your arm that you can inflate or deflate at will. The important point is to keep the circles circular and not put corners on them. In this way, you can control the space between yourself and your opponent and only let them in closer if you choose to.

- *Yield and control.* Remember that 'yielding to an incoming attack' is not the same as having your structural defences collapsed by the attacker. Even as you melt away so that your opponent cannot find anything to push on, your structure is intact and you are in control.

- *Other circles* to consider include rolling the dantien and redirecting incoming forces in a circular manner that first yields and then circles the force and returns it into the opponent. A vertical circle can be very effective when delivering a push to uproot an opponent, for example, but with practice, you will be able to circle energies in any direction you choose and you can combine them in different ways. For example, if you use a horizontal circle so that your opponent's push rolls off the 'rim of the wheel' you can follow this by taking their force downwards and return it to them diagonally upwards to uproot them. The power is generated through the whole body via the vertical rolling of the dantien. In this way the structural circles allow you to play with loops and spirals and to issue linear forces as tangents from these curves.

- *The jin circle.* Single, fixed-step push hands is the ideal training ground in which to explore the different types of jin. You first of all learn to keep your touch light and sensitive. In some schools, students and teachers enjoy this bit so much that they not only spend a disproportionate amount of time on this aspect but some even claim that push hands is just a sensitivity exercise and there is nothing 'martial' about it. We assume that you are looking to use push hands as it was intended, to help you to learn to fight, and you will therefore enjoy exploring the full circle of jins, including sticking, following, neutralising, diverting, redirecting and issuing energy, so that your defensive moves can lead naturally into a counter attack in order to unbalance your opponent.

Ultimately, you will need to progress from the very cooperative circular push hands drill and introduce a slightly more competitive element, under the supervision of your teacher, still only using one hand, with each person able to break or re-establish arm contact so that you can reach the partner's body with a well-timed push or prevent them from reaching yours. You can also practice using roll backs occasionally to divert your partner into the void, rather than returning a push as you do in the standard drill. All of these skills will be useful when you progress to the next stage - double push hands.

Double Fixed Step Push Hands

This is a progression from the single fixed-step push hands. The feet remain still but two hands can now be used for defence and attack; the objective being to uproot, destabilise and knock over the opponent while maintaining your own balance.

There are many choreographed drills that you can practice with your partner to begin with. Different styles tend to have their own favourite drills. Some of the Yang Style drills can be seen on our YouTube video on Pushing Hands. These train useful reflexes and may lead to increased sensitivity and valuable insights. However, you may wish to progress beyond these routines and introduce a competitive element. Actual blows such as punches and percussive palm or elbow strikes are not allowed. Pushes, presses, roll-backs, splitting, tilting, wrapping and plucking are among the many useful techniques still available to you.

The keys to mastery of this skill are:

- Everything you learned in single, fixed step pushing hands, plus:

- Protect your elbow

- Control your opponent's elbow

In competitions, it is usual to begin by making contact with your partner with the back of your right wrist touching theirs, as in single fixed step, and your other hand touching their elbow. Usually after three horizontal circles, the fight begins. This circling, if it happens, is usually very quick and it is easy to be caught unawares as your opponent comes at you, so you need to be ready for anything while still remaining relaxed and in control. 'Easier said than done!' you may rightly think - which is why lengthy practice of everything you have read about in previous sections is so important and why push hands competitions are so useful in testing your ability to keep calm and use your skills in a crisis.

Again, it all comes down to understanding the jin circle and practicing until all of its component skills become one smooth process which is natural and spontaneous. To recap the ingredients:

Intercept (make contact)

Adhere (attach)

Stick (stay attached)

Listen (sense everything)

Interpret (pay attention and intuitively understand what you are feeling)

Entice (if appropriate)

Receive (allow yourself to follow the incoming force without any resistance)

Neutralise (redirect)

Seize (take control)

Issue (launch your attack)

To be able to listen, you have to be able to let go of all muscular tension or force, relax and sink down into your legs and free up the waist. Your mind needs to be calm and resting in the present moment.

When you are relaxed and sunk down (while still remaining 'primed' - maintaining your peng jin or ward-off energy throughout your body), the opponent's force has nothing to push against or take hold of, which confuses them and disrupts their stability so that you can easily neutralise their attack. You can even entice them into this unstable position by creating the appearance of vulnerability.

With good timing, you can then take advantage of the opportunity in that moment to redirect the opponent's incoming energy. You can then either draw them to the side and past you so that they now have their back to you, at which point you can issue your own energy to assist them past you, perhaps onto the floor, or you might choose to uproot them and bounce them backwards as if they ran into a rubber ball.

In a real fight, you might use a full blast of explosive energy at this point but in a friendly push hands or sensing hands meeting it is enough to cause your partner to become off-balance and aware that you could take it further if you chose to. In this way, respectful practice benefits both partners and presents useful lessons for both without the need to humiliate or injure each other.

Seizing is taking control of your opponent, usually by softly making contact with moveable joints such as the wrist, elbow or shoulder. It is not the same as grabbing! We control the elbow and wrist during a roll back, for example. We might also lift the elbow and completely destabilise an opponent's posture so that we can easily knock them over. To avoid this happening to you, never allow an opponent to get control of your wrist, elbow or shoulder. If you so much as feel their intention to touch those parts, your whole body responds:

107

If they go for an elbow, you might, for example, pull the elbow in and down, sink into your legs and turn your waist so that they can no longer seize your elbow. It may also be possible to exploit the moment of their failed attempt. By dropping, you will be lower and, as you rise back up, you can issue peng jin to unbalance them.

If they try to grab your wrist, you might spiral your arm so that it becomes as slippery as an eel and, rather than just rest content that your arm is still free, stick to them and use your coiling surge to roll-back or drill forward.

Gently 'rolling' a shoulder can undo an attempt to control it.

Once you wriggle out of whatever attempt was made to grab you, don't just stop and wait for them to try something else; continue on through with your own counter-manoeuvre before they have a chance to notice what's happening.

As well as controlling an opponent's joints from the outside of an arm, it is also possible to seize and control the biceps, elbows and forearms from the inside by splitting an incoming double-handed push, for example. By then dropping one arm and raising the other, you may be able to tilt them off-balance and follow through with a push to help them on their way.

Double fixed step push hands/sensing hands can help you to learn a huge amount about the Tai Chi fighting principles. As well as appropriate timing, you can learn how far to take an opponent without losing your ability to stick to them and without over-committing yourself in any direction and thereby losing your own stability, which would allow your opponent an opportunity to sense your vulnerability and launch a counter-attack before you have a chance to seize or issue.

There are many different drills to train fixed-step pushing or sensing hands. In our school, we divide these drills into categories of square, circle and triangle or wedge; each teaching how to respond to different incoming forces or energies.

Avoid double-weightedness

The concept of double-weightedness is quite a controversial subject since there are different interpretations of what it means.

The first, and possibly the most popular, interpretation is the mistake of having your weight evenly distributed between both your legs so that you become stuck in one place and are unable to move freely in response to your opponent. Clearly, this is not a good position to be in, except at the very beginning or end of a Tai Chi sequence or in a stationary qigong posture. All the way through any Tai Chi sequence, the weight constantly shifts from one leg to the other without stopping in the middle in this double-weighted position.

However, it is worth remembering that the body can avoid double-weightedness by moving forwards and backwards and therefore does not need to constantly shift from side to side as well. In a forward stance, trying to include some side to side motion can be counter-productive and get you even more stuck.

When practitioners try to avoid the equal distribution of weight between the feet at all costs, they tend to go to the opposite extreme and 'throw their hips out' in their forward stances or back stances, with all their weight planted diagonally into a corner; sometimes even raising the front toes or back heel off the floor. This error not only makes it easier for an opponent to knock them over, it also prevents them from being able to use their waist and dantien effectively and prevents proper sinking and rooting. In other words, they are no longer actually doing Tai Chi!

Moving Step Push Hands

When you are skilled at fixed-step push hands, there will eventually come a time when you are finally allowed to move your feet!

It may seem obvious that, in a real fight, you don't actually have to stand still but, when people have been practicing fixed step for years, remembering to move the legs can be a bit of a challenge. To help to accustom you to the idea of actually walking around a bit, there are innumerable two-person drills that you can practice with a partner which involve moving the feet, including Seven Stars Stepping, Nine-Palace Stepping and various Da Lu exercises and prescribed San Shou routines (not to be confused with the free-fighting San Shou described below.)

The jump from fixed to moving step can be so great that when people begin to do it competitively, everything they know about Tai Chi can evaporate from their heads and they suddenly find themselves locked together in what tends to look more like judo or sumo wrestling.

It takes a huge amount of practice to become so confident that you are able to remain relaxed and draw upon your Tai Chi skills while engaging with a partner in a situation where both of you can move around freely in any direction.

When you do begin to explore this with various partners, you will find that some skills that worked brilliantly at fixed step range may be ineffective against someone who has longer arms and is able to move further away, or against someone who keeps coming closer than you are used to and uses grappling techniques to throw you onto the floor.

You can then see that the vital learning objective at this stage is to master the ranges: the distances between yourself and your opponent.

Ranges

Your ideal range and the style of Tai Chi you practice will be largely determined by your height and build. You can only find what works best for you by trial and error so, as always, practice is better than any amount of written advice we can offer but, for what it's worth, here are a few tips based on our own experience over the years.

Strategies that we have found to work at various ranges:

- Tilt

- Circle

- Bounce

- Bump

- Throw

- Sweep

- Body lock

These techniques can be used after the initial ward-off at the start of the bout has been split, or if one or both people chose not to maintain their ward-off.

Long Range - Tilt

When an opponent takes hold of your upper arms with their own arms firm like a bull with long horns, you may have an opportunity to unbalance them by tilting. This does not mean leaning sideways, it means remaining upright and balanced while applying downwards pressure to one arm and upward pressure to the other, thus tipping them sideways without losing your own equilibrium. This only works if their arms are stiff. If they are more relaxed, they will probably be closer to you and their arms will be too flexible to succumb to tilt, in which case we can make good use of circling.

Medium Range – Circle

At the medium range, which is the range at which fixed step push hands takes place, you are able to stick to your opponent's arms in a relaxed manner, rolling and circling as in Cloud Hands (Yun Shou), where the arms circle outwards, or its opposite (Rou Shou or 'soft hands'), where they roll inwards. You might also use a combination of both in which both arms draw circles in the same direction, one after the other, in a wrapping or threading action.

This rolling, wriggling action is not an end in itself; it is just a way of preventing an opponent from gaining an advantage by gripping your wrist or arm or controlling your elbow or shoulder.

At the same time, you remain conscious of protecting your centre line and aware of your opponent's centre. You adhere, stick, listen, interpret, receive, neutralise, seize and issue, as always, and take advantage of opportunities the opponent creates for you to unbalance them.

You might issue your energy via a push through the centre-line, but at this range, one of the most effective types of push is one that comes off the rim of a circle. This is similar to tilting but softer and at a closer range. Instead of only lifting and pressing the opponent's arms, you may be able to apply the circle to the opponent's whole body as your ascending arm takes control of their shoulder and tips them sideways. This is a movement familiar to anyone who practices the 48 step combined Taiji form and it is reminiscent of the way a cricket spin bowler launches a ball, but without lifting your arm too far or involving your shoulder in the movement. Keep your arm soft, your shoulders down, and let the elbow be the centre of the circle. This movement also works well at close range.

Close Range – Bounce and Roll-back

When an opponent moves in closer, you can use close-range fa jin to bounce them away. This may be via a double-handed push or a press or ward-off. You become like a rubber ball which has two types of strength: bounce and spin. From the point of view of the ball, no effort is required; it just absorbs and gives back or it spins on its vertical axis. The opponent is then either uprooted and repelled backwards or is led into a 'funnel' to the side and rear of where you are standing, as in a roll-back, so that you are now behind them and can easily knock them over or take them to the floor.

Bouncing from the rim of the circle or turning to deflect their force with a roll-back are the most common techniques here, but there are variations. For example, if an opponent splits your ward-off and applies downward pressure to your arms; as their push comes in, allow them to apply pressure to your arms and then bounce them back with your arms forming a wedge, as in play guitar. 'Receiving is releasing'. This is a high level skill and requires expert timing.

Grappling Range – Bump and Throw

When an opponent is so close that their body is right up against yours, you can bring your shoulder round to 'bump' them and issue jin via a shoulder strike or shoulder press. Your circling can now be used to throw them onto the floor

If they try to do the same to you, you may be able to put your arms around them and apply a body lock or bear hug so that they are unable to take you down without going down with you.

In a Tai Chi competition, that's where it ends, but in your training, it is a good idea to practice what you would do if the fight goes to the ground. Ground fighting is a subject of its own. The idea is that Tai Chi makes you so well balanced that the fight never goes to the ground. However, it is well worth gaining some practice in this type of combat, just in case you were to find yourself in this predicament in real life. At the very least, practice getting down onto the floor and up again lots of times to make sure that you are able to get back onto your feet, whatever your age, if at all possible. Ideally do this with your hands in front of you to protect yourself.

If your opponent tries to put a body lock (or bear hug) on you and you feel that there is no escape because they have come in too fast, then you also need to apply a body lock to them, but make sure that your body lock is lower than theirs. If their arms are around your chest, yours will go around their waist and hips. This gives you a lower centre of gravity so that you are able to pull them in, use your shoulder and squeeze them as hard as possible, which starts to bend their back and cause them to lose their balance so that you can either pick them up and throw them or step behind their feet, trip them up and land on top of them.

If at any point, the opponent disengages and rushes in at you again with the intention of applying a body lock, you might decide to either ward-off, or apply double biceps control, or drop lower as they come into range and bump them back with a shoulder strike, hitting them square in the centre line of the chest area or, if you are shorter, the abdomen. If you mistime your shoulder bump and they manage to get a half body-lock on you, then turn and throw them by allowing the side of your body they are pressing against to yield while your other arm comes around to knock them over and take them to the floor. If your throw is unsuccessful, continue to turn towards them and push them away from you.

Sweeping the legs can be used at various ranges to assist in unbalancing an opponent but it is important not to destroy your own root in the attempt. Sweeps work best just inside circling range when control is being applied to your arms and you use their focus on control as an opportunity to break their root while they are distracted.

San Shou

San Shou (or San Da) is an opportunity to test your skills in a full-contact fight. Unlike push hands, you can kick and punch as well as using pushes and throws. For this reason, you can wear protective items such as shin guards, groin guard, gum shield and boxing gloves and even body armour.

Having said that, you still can't fully test the kind of Tai Chi skills you would need the most in a real fight. The rules do not allow blows to the neck or groin. In San Shou, boxing gloves are compulsory and they prevent you from using open palm strikes.

What usually happens in San Shou competitions is that the whole thing turns into a kick boxing match, though occasionally skilled Tai

115

Chi practitioners will get in close and use their Tai Chi skills instead of just kicking and punching. We have heard people say that it is impossible to use any of the movements from the Tai Chi forms in a San Shou competition and that it has to be more of a kick boxing fight. We feel that this undervalues Tai Chi as a martial art and we can attest to the fact that it is possible to use Tai Chi moves in such competitions if you have practiced the skills enough and are able to remain calm enough to use those skills, rather than tensing up and relying on ordinary muscular effort.

People do sometimes sustain injuries in these competitions but the safety of contestants is a major consideration.

Competitions

Tai Chi is often seen as a non-competitive pursuit. Although this is obviously not true, when you consider the number of local and international competitions both inside and outside China, it can give that impression, especially in the West, where most people practice it only for their health and well-being and have no interest in fighting. The principles of Tai Chi are all about balance and going with the flow so, in general, most of us do tend to be pretty laid back and peace-loving types who have no desire to glorify ourselves at other people's expense.

The down side of any competition is that someone has to lose and even the winners can end up with a reputation to maintain that's more of a burden than a pedestal to climb upon (there will always be someone who wants to knock you off it). These are good arguments and there are many highly-skilled Tai Chi practitioners and instructors who never compete, for these and other ethical reasons.

However, our purpose in writing this book is to enable you to equip yourself with skills that may increase your chances of survival in a potentially hostile world, and competitions can be useful to you in the process of acquiring and testing these skills. Competitions can be seen as a bridge between class-based practice and a real-life conflict situation.

We have provided many examples of students who have actually been attacked on the street and have prevailed by using their Tai Chi skills. Most of these have been elderly people who have never participated in any kind of partner work; simply learning their hand forms was sufficient to provide them with unconscious skills that came to their aid in a crisis. Then again, as we have seen, practicing push hands with a range of partners in class, under the supervision of your teacher, can be extremely beneficial in further developing your skills and understanding of the art.

An even greater challenge is to enter a competition, where you will be testing your skills against people you never met before who have trained with different instructors. This is about as close as you can get to a real-life fight without deliberately going out of your way to look for trouble! (Not recommended.)

The stress of competitions also helps you to get used to experiencing the effects of hormones such as adrenalin in a setting which is less dangerous than an encounter with a real life assailant.

In the following section, we will offer a few tips and insights into what to expect in competitions, based on the experiences of our own fighters in national and international events.

What to expect in competitions

If you are thinking about having a go at a competition, we would recommend that you begin by going along to one or two as a spectator to see what you are letting yourself in for! If you then want to go ahead, start with small local competitions before progressing to larger events.

The competitions may include hand forms, weapons forms, pushing hands (fixed step and moving step) and free fighting (San Shou/San Da). You would be well advised to start with the push hands and only progress to San Shou when you have gained a lot of experience in competitions and trained for full contact fighting.

Preparing for the event

If watching from the side-lines doesn't put you off and you feel that you are ready to have a go, make sure that you get a copy of the rules of the particular competition you are entering well in advance of the advent and read these very carefully so that you have time to train with those rules in mind, though do also be aware that there can be changes to these on the day!

You can download a set of international competition rules from the website of the British Council for Chinese Martial Arts (www.bccma.com) to give you an idea of what is normally expected, but do bear in mind that the organisers of different events may have different requirements and these may change from year to year, so you need to contact the organisers of the event you are entering to obtain a copy of their current regulations.

Train hard, train smart, fight easy! It's no good having a lot of skill if you are so unfit you can't last a round against someone of equivalent skills, and it's no good being fighting fit if you don't know how to use Tai Chi. Like the Yin and the Yang, you need a balanced approach to your training.

On the day – the realities of competition

There will probably be some kind of dress code. You will be expected to have the right clothing and any necessary equipment with you. You need to know whether you will be expected to wear long trousers or shorts, a vest or a T shirt (in some cases you need to have T shirts of appropriate colours while in others you will be provided with a coloured sash so that the referee and judges can identify which person scores the points in a bout.) In San Shou you will need a gum shield, head guard, body armour and groin guard and an appropriate pair of boxing gloves.

There will normally be weight categories and you will need to weigh in and be registered at the start of the competition. If your weight is different to the weight category you entered on your application form, you can be disqualified and have to re-register in a different category and pay an additional fee.

If there are insufficient people in a particular weight category on the day, then different weight categories may be combined or even scrapped altogether. This can be particularly challenging if you have starved yourself for weeks to get into a particular category only to find that the competition is now 'open weight' and you are up against someone twice your size or even someone of the opposite gender!

Be prepared for the unexpected and be prepared for the sheer boredom of sitting around for hours waiting for your turn while also attempting to remain 'warmed up' and physically and mentally prepared to fight.

Occasionally, you may also need to be ready to plunge straight into the next round after a heavy bout, with little or no time to get your breath back in between.

Rules of Push Hands

In fixed step, the only movement of the feet allowed is the raising of the front toes. Any other movement of the front or back foot is not allowed. This is double fixed step push hands where you are free to use both hands. We have not come across a competition with a single-handed push hands category. You begin by bowing to your opponent and facing them with your right foot forward, making contact with your partner's forearm at wrist and elbow.

Points are awarded to you if your partner moves any part of a foot, other than the toes of the front foot, or takes a step in any direction (one point) or two steps (two points) or touches the floor with any part of the body above the foot (three points). If you both fall over, no points are awarded in most competitions we know. In some competitions, if you manage to throw your opponent using your ward off or roll back in such a way that both their feet leave the floor, you score four points.

Moving step push hands takes place within a defined area, which could be a square or circular mat or a raised platform. Points are awarded when you unbalance your opponent, cause them to fall over or cause them to step outside the designated area.

You can also incur points against you if you infringe any other competition rules such as the dress code, showing up late, aggressive behaviour, 'unsportsmanlike' conduct, not following the instructions of the judges or using any illegal moves.

Some Examples of Prohibited Techniques

- Using your hands to lift an opponent's leg.
- Scratching the opponent with your nails.
- Use of nerve or pressure point holds.
- Attacks to the face, the back of the head or the throat.
- Attacks to the groin.
- Joint locks.
- Striking an opponent with your head, elbows or knees.
- Kicks.
- Holding or pulling of clothes or hair.
- Attacking the opponent's joints: such as knees, wrists, elbows, thumbs or fingers.
- Holding onto your opponent to prevent losing your balance.

Rules of San Shou

In San Shou, you are allowed to attack the head, trunk and thighs but you are not allowed to attack the back of the head, the neck or the groin. You can use any type of Wu Shu including any style of Tai Chi, Xing Yi, Bagua and others but you are not allowed to attack using the head, the elbow or the knee. You are not allowed to attack the head of the opponent when he or she is down, with any technique.

A complete list of the scoring criteria and International Rules of San Shou are normally available on the website of the British Council for Chinese Martial Arts (BCCMA). The list will provide you with an example of the kind of rules that might apply in most competitions. If you are seriously considering entering a competition, however, you need to get hold of a copy of the current regulations for the specific event you will be attending.

Once you have understood the rules and undergone appropriate training for the event, it is also worth considering how you might prepare yourself mentally for the challenge. In particular, you might like to consider how you will deal with emotions such as fear and anger so that you can remain relatively calm and able to focus and use your skills effectively.

Self-mastery

The practice of push hands helps you to master yourself as much or more than you learn to dominate an opponent.

Ice and water

In his excellent book The Unfettered Mind: Writings from a Zen Master to a Swordsman, Takuan Soho advises us to keep the mind fluid at all times. When the attention is focussed on the sword of the opponent, the mind is like ice and our responses are slow, but when it is fluid, the mind is like water, the opponent's weapon becomes our own and we are able to take it from him.

Bruce Lee advised us to be aware of the opponent's whole body energy, by which he meant exactly what Takuan Soho was referring to: being present in the moment with all your senses open and alert to everything about your opponent and your surroundings so that you are not caught up in the blinkered, tunnel vision of a trance state. We will be saying much more about this in a moment (Step 6).

Dealing with fear

We have already seen how the fight or flight response can help us to fight, run away or sometimes freeze. In a competition, the first option is the one we want. Adrenalin will almost certainly be present but it can be a good thing in that it gives us more than our normal strength and speed, as long as we don't allow our anxiety to either paralyse us or generate tension in the body that prevents us from using our martial skills, which rely on relaxation.

The key to coping in situations like this is to mentally step back from our thoughts and find the quiet space underlying everything. This ability can be trained by regular meditation practice and also by the mindful practice of your Tai Chi forms. When we rest in Wu Chi, we are able to remain calm and do what needs to be done at that moment without the brain interfering by dreaming up worst case scenarios and 'what-if's, which fear and anxiety thrive on.

Take your time on each out breath while you are waiting for your turn in the ring. Breathing out more slowly than you breathe in stimulates the parasympathetic nervous system and triggers the relaxation response.

It may also help to view each bout as an interesting learning experience for both participants. Feel what is happening with your opponent and respond accordingly. See what works and what doesn't. Winning or losing is kind of irrelevant. In years to come, few will remember the names of all the medallists but you will remember the lessons you learned that contributed to your development as a Tai Chi practitioner and teacher.

In general, we recommend that, if you do decide to enter a competition, you leave your ego at the door and be prepared to learn more from your losses than from your victories. In our own experience, being knocked down many times has taught us the most about how to stand up. If you lose a fight, don't lose the lesson.

Dealing with anger

If you 'lose it' and react blindly to a real or imagined insult, or even if you get angry with yourself for making a 'stupid mistake', you are no longer in control of the situation and you will be too tense to use anything but brute force in the fight.

All the posturing, 'psyching each other out' and generally being unpleasant to each other before boxing matches is just an act designed for the media. Real hostility cripples a fighter by putting them in their emotional brain, locking them into a trance state and making all their hard-won martial arts skills useless.

Don't let yourself get into eyeballing each other; rest your gaze lightly on their upper chest and maintain your all-round awareness. Stay sunk, rooted and relaxed.

Smile. You can't be angry when you're laughing.

We have seen that psychology plays an important role in pushing hands competitions; it is crucial when you are out on the street. The next Chapter will explore in detail how human minds work - your own and those of any potential criminals out there - so that you are better equipped to deal with an assailant or, preferably, to do everything you can to avoid trouble in the first place.

Step 6

Avoid Trouble

'The physical techniques of Self Protection are worthless without a correct attitude to personal security. The basis of good security is 'Constant Awareness'.'

The British Combat Association

All the skills that you have learned so far, in class-based exercises and possibly competitions, are ultimately practiced as preparation for real life.

Recently, as one of us was leaving a building where she had been teaching, she paused to get her car keys out of her bag, mentioning to the people she was with that, as a martial artist, she needed to practice what she preached and make sure she had the keys in her hand before going out into the car park.

Why, they asked, would a martial artist need to have their keys in their hand? She explained that it was dark, and she didn't want to be rummaging in her bag when she got to her car and, in any case, a bunch of keys could be a good weapon.

"But that's not martial arts!" they said. "It's just self-protection!"

Clearly, it had never occurred to them that martial arts is all about self-protection!

We were so astonished that we spent a couple of weeks discussing the subject with everyone we knew. We discovered that, in most people's minds, martial arts and self-protection are two entirely different subjects. Self-protection, apparently, is 'just common sense' while martial arts are all about 'esoteric wisdom and cool, kick-ass moves!'

Yet learning a martial art is not just about learning how to fight; it's about staying alive and keeping safe, and that's largely a result of taking precautions that help you to avoid dangerous situations in the first place.

Self-defence is possibly better defined as: 'What you have to do when all your Self-Protection methods have failed.'

When it comes to potentially life-threatening emergencies, an actual fight is a last resort.

The principles of self-protection come under the two broad headings of:

- How to avoid getting into dire situations, if possible (Step 6)

  and

- How to be prepared for any unpleasantness, if that becomes unavoidable (Step 7)

Both of these depend mostly on an understanding of how human minds work: yours and those of the various villains who walk among us. And walk among us they do! Though it is not our intention to induce in you a state of hyper-alertness, anxiety and paranoia - quite the opposite actually - we will be honest about the kind of risks that exist in our society in the belief that a well-informed, street-wise, awake individual has a better chance of survival than someone whose trusting innocence or general lack of awareness makes them easy prey for a predator.

While we will focus largely on avoiding risky public settings, it is worth remembering that, statistically, according to the UK Health and Safety at Work Executive and The Office for National Statistics, there is a much higher risk of being attacked by someone you already know, at home or at work, than by a stranger on the street. Though it's difficult to put a figure on it because of the number of such crimes that may go unreported, many people, especially children and women but also men, suffer violence in their own home. Whatever the moral ground we choose to make our stand on, none of us can be absolutely sure that we will never need to fight for our survival or to protect our loved ones, wherever we live in this world. For some people, that struggle is their day to day reality.

It concerns us that martial arts classes are often viewed as the exclusive domain of young, fit people, mostly male; yet studies show that armed robbers are more likely to target women over sixty. For people in this age group, Tai Chi may be more accessible than other martial arts. Even if their primary aim is to improve their health and fitness, their Tai Chi training may also equip them with the knowledge and skills they need to protect themselves.

Whatever your age and gender, avoiding trouble, though not always possible, is certainly preferable to dealing with it. In this chapter, we will look at how to lower the risk to yourself and others by developing a greater awareness of yourself and the people around you.

Self-awareness

If you only ever learn one habit from practicing Tai Chi, let it be an upright and 'noble' posture. As we have seen throughout the rest of this book, an upright spine and a level gaze are the keys to accessing all the high-level martial skills of Tai Chi but the importance of this posture is even more fundamental than that: it may reduce your chances of being attacked in the first place!

It is important to understand, before you read on, that we are not in any way suggesting that a violent crime is the fault of the victim. Criminals are responsible for the crimes they commit, however much they might try to justify their actions by claiming that their victims 'asked for it'. What we are doing here is looking at some very interesting research that we believe everyone should know about if this knowledge can help to prevent them from becoming victims of violent crime.

In a now famous study by Betty Grayson and Morris I. Stein in 1981, a group of criminals were asked to watch a video of people walking down a street. Unaware that they were being observed, the criminals immediately began to identify which of the people they would have targeted for violent crimes, including robbery, rape and murder. Their responses were unexpected.

Outweighing any preference for victims of a particular age, height, race or gender, the main characteristic that made people stand out as potential targets was their way of standing and moving. Like lions prowling the edges of a herd of wildebeest on the plains of Africa, these predators were assessing the likelihood that each potential victim would be able to put up a fight!

Look at the way you normally stand and walk. Observe yourself in a full-length mirror or ask a friend to video you if that helps. Look at the position of your spine and your head. Is your back straight or curved? Are you looking down at the floor most of the time with your head bowed? Do you normally walk with your shoulders back, chest out and nose in the air? Or are your shoulders hunched like a Rottweiler about to attack?

It might come as no surprise to learn that predators prey on the weak and the vulnerable but the research also showed that apparent vulnerability was judged more by actions than by size.

Submissive posture

People who shuffled down the street with their heads down were the most likely to be seen as potential victims. The researchers found that even large men, if they behaved in this way, were more likely to be targeted than petite women who were upright and alert! Even the way women dressed was less important than the way they carried themselves, which is again the opposite of what we might expect.

Other researchers have found that women covered from neck to toe who look fearful and submissive are more likely to become targets of sexual assault than those who some might consider to be 'provocatively dressed' yet appear alert and confident (in Western culture at least – though the assailant may have religious beliefs that make the opposite true). Rapists, apparently, are often more concerned with control and domination than sexual desire.

Military or confrontational postures

The military stance, on the other hand, is not necessarily much better. Criminals often see themselves as victims of society and carry a grudge against anyone who seems well-off and arrogant. If you are completely honest, have you never felt the urge to deck some smug so-and-so on the chin? And of course if you go around like a Rottweiler looking for trouble, someone might eventually oblige...

Tai Chi posture

When you see Tai Chi performed well, the spine will be straight and the head will be upright as if suspended from above by an invisible thread. The shoulders will be dropped but not stooped. The gaze will be level and calm. The whole appearance will be of relaxed confidence and control; a kind of effortless grace, combined with hidden reserves of power, like a tiger prowling through a forest.

All of this is necessary for Tai Chi to work properly. Looking up or down alters the alignment of the vertebrae so that you are unable to use your waist and dantien properly and therefore cannot access your internal power. Tension leads to stiffness, which scuppers the whole thing.

Even when you are not performing a Tai Chi sequence, if you stand and walk like a Tai Chi person, you will look like someone who knows how to handle yourself. This is not necessarily an illusion, whatever your age, gender or stature. Several of our elderly students have successfully defended themselves against muggers with a Tai Chi push or roll back, and many a strong and youthful challenger has been tossed away like a rag doll by one of the old men who practice Push Hands in the parks of Beijing. If you want your posture to give out a message to would-be assailants, let it be a quietly confident: 'Don't mess with me!'

Another aspect of self-awareness is to understand how the mind works so that you can recognise your own mental states and know what to do about them.

Self-control

There is a vital skill that is common to all martial arts, and that is self-mastery. No amount of martial training will be of any use to you if you are standing paralysed with fear or so angry that you totally lose the plot and start saying or doing stupid things that you will regret later on.

Self-control may be required not only in an encounter with an aggressive drunk or a homicidal maniac but also in some fairly ordinary situations. Supposing you found yourself sitting in the back of a police car on your way to a wedding. The police have pulled you over because their number plate recognition software has identified you as having no vehicle insurance. It's the weekend and it takes a whole hour for them to verify your claim that you paid your renewal premium a month ago. At the end of the hour, they apologise, having discovered that the insurance company has not shared their records with the central police database.

Frustrating? Yes. Upsetting that you totally missed the wedding? Very! However, the ability to mentally step back and observe your own emotional brain, and override its instinctive responses to swear or to hit someone, can perhaps save you the additional discomfort of spending time in a prison cell.

Frustration is understandable. Anger is understandable and, in some situations, unavoidable. What can make all the difference in preventing an upsetting initial predicament from escalating into a full-blown calamity is your ability to see what your mind is up to and then choose your response to the circumstances, rather than to react to them.

How the Mind Works

There are few things in the universe more complex than the human brain and, unfortunately, it doesn't come with an instruction manual! However, psychologists and neuroscientists can offer us one or two very useful tips that can help us to choose our responses to life's challenging circumstances.

If you have ever felt yourself to be 'in two minds' about something, or if someone you know seems to have 'two sides to them': a bit of a 'Jekyll and Hyde', this is not at all surprising. A natural feature of the human brain is that we tend to think in different ways, depending on whether we are feeling calm or emotionally aroused.

When we are calm, we can use the higher cortex or frontal lobes of the brain, which is where all our best reasoning skills lie. When we are over-emotional, however, our access to these higher processes is cut off, leaving us to use a more primitive area of the brain, the limbic system, to do our thinking for us.

Effectively, we have an 'emotional brain' and a 'rational brain' and, to have any chance of using the latter, we need to calm down. That's why it's generally best to have a good night's sleep before writing an angry letter, or to take a walk around the block before saying something we might later regret.

There's a good reason for having 'two minds': the fight or flight response. Evolution has programmed us to respond instantly to a life-threatening situation. If a train is hurtling towards you, you simply don't have time to stand around calculating its incoming velocity and working out a suitable avoidance strategy, so your body just leaps itself out of the way and lets your rational brain catch up later.

This ability has no doubt contributed to the survival of our species but it is not always quite so helpful. There are times when we have to keep a hot temper in check or go outside our comfort zone to do an essential job that we find a bit scary. From rescuing someone from a burning building to refraining from punching the guy in the bar who insulted us, there are times when we need to keep calm in a crisis or to control our anger.

What can help is the knowledge that, when we respond to some external situation, the feeling arises before the thought, so there's nothing to be gained from beating yourself up for being scared or angry. What matters is what you choose to do about it once you realise that's how you're feeling.

Here's how the brain works:

When we notice what's going on around us, information from our senses goes into our brain via two walnut-sized areas called the amygdalae. These act like a couple of security guards on the door. They have the ID details of everything that came through previously and they are trained to tell the difference between the good stuff and the potentially harmful stuff. They then do the mental equivalent of sticking a post-it note on the incoming information, expressing their initial feelings about it, before passing it on to the limbic system - the brain's secretary.

If the incoming information is that all is well and there's something interesting or helpful going on here, the secretary passes it on to the boss upstairs in the higher cortex. If, on the other hand, the information is that there's a bus coming towards us at a rather alarming rate, the secretary doesn't have time to let the boss know and so just sorts it out then and there by triggering the release of emergency hormones such as adrenalin and getting the body out of danger fast.

Adrenalin might not be the nicest hormone on the block - most people don't particularly enjoy the panting lungs, the knotted stomach or the heart palpitations - but these do serve a useful purpose in a crisis. We breathe faster to get oxygen into our blood, which the heart then pumps extra-quickly to the muscles and the brain, along with extra sugar for energy, so that we can run, fight, lift a car off an injured casualty, deliver a pre-emptive strike or leap over a wall in order to escape the attentions of a villain!

In less extreme situations, the boss might just get a peek at what's going on and decide to intervene and calm everything down so that a more considered response is possible.

As well as the options of fight or flight, there is a third possibility: in some situations, people freeze. In terms of our evolutionary survival, this might seem to be the least helpful of all our inbuilt responses, yet even this may have its uses.

A gazelle on the plains of Africa may dangle, apparently lifeless, from the jaws of a cheetah as it is dragged away to become dinner. This freeze response, however, allows it to restore its energy. The cheetah, exhausted from the chase and all that gazelle-dragging, settles down to get her breath back, letting go of the seemingly dead gazelle, who now makes a startling recovery and bounds away with a bit of a sore neck but still alive.

The point here is that, once an opportunity for escape presented itself, the gazelle didn't hang around and wait to be eaten. Timing, sometimes, is everything.

In Tai Chi, we learn to conserve our energy, relaxing until there is an opening to strike, or to flee. When we strike, we give it everything we have, and if there's some residual adrenalin around to fuel that action, so much the better.

How to Calm Down

From working with convicted felons in a large prison, we discovered that a majority had committed crimes while they were emotionally wound up and 'couldn't think straight'. Many said that if they had learned Tai Chi, Qigong or meditation years ago, their lives may have gone down very different paths. Those who attended Tai Chi classes during their stay in prison said that they felt much calmer and less inclined to be violent. They felt that they now had more options of how to think and feel rather than just 'getting stuck in!'

There are some useful tricks you can learn to help you to get out of your emotional brain.

1. Seven eleven breathing

The simplest method of all is to breathe out more slowly than you breathe in.

Sounds too simple? Well actually it's a biological process that always works because it stimulates a thing called the parasympathetic nervous system and triggers the Relaxation Response, which is the opposite of the Fight or Flight response. When you are breathing out more slowly than you breathe in, your body automatically switches off the adrenalin and begins to relax.

This is sometimes called 7:11 breathing - you breathe in for a count of seven and breathe out for a count of eleven - but the numbers don't matter, just take your time over the out breath.

This is an excellent way to defuse a 'panic attack' or state of anxiety.

2. Tai Chi breathing

When people are over-anxious, their breath tends to be very fast and shallow, using the top part of the lungs. As a Tai Chi practitioner, you can bring the breath all the way down to the lower abdomen, fully inflating the lower lobes of the lungs which allows you to take in more oxygen with each breath and breathe more slowly.

One of us once arrived at a Xing Yi session after running for several miles, including a final stretch uphill. She was gasping for air and couldn't even speak. Her teacher was not impressed. Apparently that was not acceptable behaviour for a Tai Chi person! Her breathless attempts to protest that it was impossible to breathe normally were met with a calm: 'Breathe from your dantien.' So she gave it a go and, after about three breaths, she was pretty much back to normal!

Calming down and breathing properly is not only a good idea if you want to think clearly, it's also essential if you want to use any of your Tai Chi skills.

While we have already talked about breathing in previous chapters, it is so important that we will recap again here the key points of how to breathe from your dantien:

Breathe in while keeping your chest down and your abdomen flat, so that your sides expand and it feels as though your back is inflating with air.

As you breathe out, let your knees soften and allow your weight to drop down into your legs and your tail bone to drop towards the floor.

At the same time, gently squeeze your pelvic floor muscles and allow your lower abdomen to lift at the front and roll inwards under your ribs by contracting your upper abdominal muscles as your lower ones relax.

If you make a 'hhwwwaaaa' sound as you breathe out, you will find that this movement happens naturally.

After a bit of practice, you can simply imagine the air or energy coming in through your nose and out through a point about an inch below your navel as your lower abdomen rotates like a football.

If you are still unsure about what we mean, there is a whole chapter on Tai Chi breathing, with useful exercises to help you to develop this skill, in our previous book: *How to Move Towards Tai Chi Mastery: 7 Practical Steps to Improve Your Forms and Access your Internal Power.*

3. Stepping back and taking a wider view

The emotional brain is very primitive and highly illogical. It thinks in very simple, black and white terms such as: 'He's wrong; I'm right!' There are no shades of grey in the middle! It also tends to over-generalise. A clear sign that you are in your emotional brain is when you start using words like 'always', 'everything' and 'everywhere':

'It always happens to me!' 'Everything has gone wrong!' 'The whole world is messed up!'

This 'catastrophic thinking' can make you feel, speak and act like a victim, either by over-reacting or by giving up and becoming submissive. Calming down puts you back in control of your thoughts and actions and allows you to gain a clearer perspective of what is going on and what to do about it.

You may then have a chance to take control of the situation by being assertive rather than passive or aggressive.

The ability to mentally step back and take a wider view is therefore invaluable. In an argument, just by considering what an onlooker would see, we can begin to defuse the anger and allow the rational brain to get a look in.

Having said this, some people act more aggressively when they know other people are watching and actually enjoy 'playing to the audience' as if they somehow expect sympathy or praise from onlookers. Removing the audience brings their 'performance' to an end. Be aware of this possibility and make sure that you are not doing it yourself!

Stepping back from your own thoughts and realising that you are in your emotional brain allows you to take action to calm yourself down. This is a skill that is developed by the practice of meditation and mindfulness: being in the moment, right here and now, with your attention open in all directions. The overall calming effect of these practices can also make you less likely to become over-emotional in the first place.

However, it is important to mention again here that, in an extreme emergency, such as the point at which you realise that someone is holding a knife against your ribs, there is usually a massive release of adrenalin that can temporarily overwhelm you. In such a situation, it is unlikely that you will be able to maintain absolute calm in the face of your possibly impending demise but there is a chance that the mental habit of stepping back and detaching from your emotions will allow you to calm down sufficiently to use the adrenalin to fight or to get out of there fast. Potentially, you may even be able to think more clearly and see what to do, as extra sugar and oxygen is delivered to your brain.

The cold state

An angry person is often described as being hot-tempered and it brings to mind the picture of someone with a red face, but there may be times when anger becomes such deep outrage that we become intensely calm and the colour drains from our cheeks. It is not a pleasant type of calm, however. The world around you can seem quite unreal and you may not be doing very much thinking at all. The safest thing to do at such times is to remove yourself from the situation. If you are faced with a person who is in this condition, watch out!

It is also worth mentioning here that psychopaths are not affected by emotions in the way we have described above. They lack empathy for others and, while they may seem to be very courteous and charismatic, they may be very cold and unfeeling inside. They really don't care about how anyone else feels, which is how they often manage to become very successful in business. It is estimated that about one percent of the global population - around seventy million people - are psychopaths! Only a few might be cold-blooded killers but very many of them end up running banks, corporations and countries. If this topic interests you, Jon Ronson's book: *The Psychopath Test* makes fascinating reading.

Situation-awareness

We can't avoid all risk. What we are looking at here is how to attempt to avoid unnecessary risk, or how to minimise it, by being aware of how criminals operate and taking a few precautions.

Unless someone is specifically and determinedly targeting you, in which case you need police protection and perhaps a new identity, there is much you can do to avoid some of the potential risks inherent in our society. Most of them will appear to be common sense; things you have already picked up from experience or just instinctively know. Let's take a few obvious examples:

Car Parks

Car parks are a good case in point. Apart from being a favourite haunt of beggars and muggers, they are also a popular place for abductions and worse. Although we might be on our guard if we were in a deserted underground car park at night, it's important to know that these situations can take place during the daytime and with other people around.

A couple of years ago, a nurse went out to her car in broad daylight. She got behind the wheel but reached down to pick up a water bottle that she had dropped on the floor. At that point, she was hit on the head by a heavy object, dragged from the car and left for dead while the perpetrator drove off. The criminal, in this case, did not look like most-people's idea of a car thief or potential murderer. He was a clean-shaven young man, wearing a smart, pin-striped suit. He may have been the only other person in the car park but his appearance would not have set alarm bells ringing in most people's minds.

In other cases, there is no would-be assailant to see, because they are hiding behind the car on the passenger side, or in another car parked next to it. Since most cars have a central locking system these days, when the driver gets in on one side, the villain gets in on the other. You might think that it would be an easy thing to simply get out again but that's not always the case. In some people, the panic response is so great that they freeze and can't move. One lady was abducted by a man who not only drove her to a distant site in order to harm her but even pulled in at a petrol station during the journey and fuelled up! Although the car was not locked, her legs were paralysed by her fear and she simply sat there while he got back in again and continued on his way.

A student of ours responded differently in a similar situation. She was driving home in broad daylight with her baby in the back seat and had pulled up at traffic lights when a man got in beside her. What his intentions were, we will never know because the lady, at that point, went ballistic; shouting, screaming, hitting him with everything she had and leaning on the hooter to attract the attention of passers-by. The man made a quick exit. Keeping your calm does not preclude acting like a psycho!

In general, if you are returning to your car, wherever you left it, whether that was in a car park, on the side of the road or even outside your house:

- Have your keys in your hand, rather than spend time rummaging through your pockets or bag. The same applies to house keys when you get home, especially at night.

- Check that there's no one on the other side.

- Get in quickly and

- Lock the door from the inside. You will have seen in countless movies how easy it is for a criminal to jump into the back of a car as it pulls up at traffic lights.

- If you need to put shopping in the boot, do it while maintaining awareness of your surroundings and don't lean into your car to rearrange your stuff.

- Be particularly vigilant if you are putting a baby or young child into the car and fastening their seat belt. Keep an all-round awareness at all times.

- If you need to return your shopping trolley to a 'trolley park', lock your car so that nobody can get into it while your back is turned. If it's dark and you are alone, just leave the trolley where it is and drive away.

Some of these tips may seem obvious, others bordering on paranoia, but we can only speculate how much grief might have been avoided if everyone did all of these things routinely. It's not an excessive anxiety response, it's as normal as a pilot carrying out pre-flight checks before he gets onto the runway.

Lonely streets and dark places

Being out on your own, especially when walking down deserted streets and especially at night, is obviously going to carry more risk than being out during the day with a group of trusted people, though, as we saw above, daylight does not always guarantee our safety. If you are out at night, or in a lonely place during the day, it's best not to walk next to a wall, trees, dumpsters, parked vans or anything else that someone can hide behind or inside, ready to jump out at you.

Criminals tend to prefer locations where there are no witnesses and victims who are not paying attention. It might seem like a good idea to have your phone out and chat to someone for company when you're in a scary place but a predator sees you as someone whose attention is distracted, making it easier for them to approach. The same principle applies to being out on the street while listening to music on headphones. You need all your senses available and all your wits about you if you want to improve the odds in your favour.

Alcohol and drugs

Excessive drinking dulls the senses and, whether you are male or female, if you get to a point where you are no longer aware of where you are, you are obviously going to be an easy target, however fit you are and however many years you have been practicing martial arts! Researchers have also found that rapists may interpret uninhibited behaviour under the influence of alcohol as sexual interest.

Alcohol, of course, is not the only potential problem. There are now drinking straws and nail varnishes that change colour if you dip them in a drink that has been spiked with a date-rape drug but it is still wise to pay attention to what you are drinking and what might have been added on its way to you.

In general, vigilance and staying sober enough to know what's going on are recommended on those nights out when you are having a good time.

Sick societies

Some societies have a 'gun culture' in which a majority of people are allowed to carry a loaded firearm, making your training in unarmed combat techniques seem a bit superfluous. However, even in such countries, there may be occasions when some of the advice given in these pages can help, particularly the psychological insights and overall awareness. Some of the research findings we will discuss next relate to armed robberies in the United States.

Carrying cash

People coming out of banks or using cash machines can be seen as targets by armed robbers.

If you are interested to find out more about the ways in which criminals select potential victims on the street, we can recommend the book: *'Armed Robbers in Action'* by Wright and Decker. This is an account of a major study in which researchers went out onto the streets of an American city to interview eighty-six people who made a living from armed robbery. Almost all of them used guns as their weapon of choice. In other countries where guns are illegal, they may be more likely to be carrying a knife.

Their main victims were other criminals, especially drug dealers, who would not be likely to go to the police. Men using prostitutes were seen as easy targets for similar reasons. Of the law-abiding citizens who were targeted, women over sixty were seen as the easiest, as they were less likely to fight back or attract attention. The main objective of the criminals, in this particular study, was to obtain cash quickly and without attracting attention.

Interestingly, they were far less interested in wealthy-looking people who might be more likely to be carrying plastic than cash. For this reason, and also because of the presence of security guards and wide roads where the police could easily chase after them, they tended to prefer quiet streets in poor, inner-city areas to glitzy shopping malls on the edge of town.

While older people may be more likely to be attacked by armed robbers, young adults are particularly likely to be targeted by drunken gangs who just don't like the look of them. In some cities, such attacks can be based on gang membership, racism or just someone's style of dress or the post code of the area they live in! These situations are hard to avoid. Indeed, it is in such situations that one of us gained a considerable amount of practical martial arts training! However, we are not suggesting that you should avoid going out altogether, only that you stay alert, be wise to some of the warning signs and know what to do if there is any trouble.

Kitchens

It's not only actual criminals who can pose a risk to your safety. Angry people can also be dangerous. In a moment we will look at some general advice about how to deal with difficult people but, still on the subject of avoiding risky situations, it's worth mentioning that you should never take a very angry person into a kitchen to make them a cup of tea! It may seem like a good idea to help them to calm down, but a kitchen is jam-pack full of weapons, including knives and boiling water! Going outside for a walk in the garden is a better idea. That way, if your efforts are unsuccessful, you have a better chance of escape. If you are inside a building, be aware of where the exits are and don't allow an angry or threatening person to get between you and the door or, if you are upstairs, the staircase.

145

People-awareness

How much notice do you take of other people around you? Have you ever walked right past a friend in the supermarket without noticing they were there until they spoke to you? Have you ever been so absorbed in what you were doing that you didn't even notice that someone was speaking to you until they tapped you on the arm?

If you answered 'yes' or 'often', then congratulations; you're human! We have a natural ability to focus our attention either internally or externally and to concentrate so fully on what we are doing or thinking that we temporarily block out everything else. That's fine in many circumstances. In fact it's often the best way to get things done. If you're writing a book or working out your finances or sitting an exam, it's great to be able to block out the sound of workmen out on the street or people chatting in the next room and give your full attention to what you are doing.

We can even perform some skills automatically, leaving our minds free to focus on something else. Concert pianists don't have to think about every single note they play, which leaves them free to feel and express the music. Experienced drivers don't need to think every time they change gear or press the brake pedal, which leaves them free to read road signs, watch out for pedestrians or compose a sonnet in their heads as they cruise down the highway. The downside is that we can become so absorbed in our musings that we miss our exit and end up adding an extra twenty miles to our journey!

Walking down the street focussed on what we're planning to have for lunch is a great skill - until we feel our bag leaving our fingers because we hadn't noticed the guy behind us.

Guy? Are all bag thieves male? Do all muggers, rapists and potential murderers fit into neat and easily recognisable categories? Would it surprise you to learn that some of the most dreadful crimes have been committed by people who looked as trustworthy and inoffensive as dear old granddad, or indeed grandma?

We heard of a woman and her toddler who were killed on the street by a kindly-looking man with white hair and beard who offered to help load shopping into the boot of her car. Everyone trusts Santa, right? Well maybe not everyone, but the fact that he fell into that kind of stereotype may have contributed to the demise of this poor mother and her child. Had the guy looked like Jack Nicholson or most-people's idea of a 'terrorist', it is highly unlikely that this woman would have agreed to let him help her with her shopping!

Sometimes we are too trusting or just too nice, and that can get us into a whole lot of trouble!

Imagine that gazelle on the plains of Africa. It grazes, listening, constantly alert. A gust of wind, an oddly shaped rock half seen from the corner of an eye, and it's already running, then slowing as it realises it was a false alarm, and it returns to grazing. A lion approaches and again the gazelle is running...it lives.

How different if the gazelle had human instincts! A lion approaches. The gazelle looks it in the face and strives to look cool. It mustn't run away. This may be a lion with good intentions and it is important not to cause offence unnecessarily, isn't it? Running away might look silly or cowardly to anyone who might be watching. Better, perhaps, just to stand around and wait to see what happens...

In a local supermarket, a lady we know was looking at some frozen peas when she became aware of another woman standing very close to her. She felt uneasy about the close proximity but didn't want to cause offence to the woman by moving away. It was only when she reached the checkout and put a hand inside her bag to take out her purse that she discovered that, not only was her purse not there but the entire bottom section of her bag was not there either. The woman had used a knife to cut off half the bag and all its contents!

Predatory criminals rely on your good nature, your reluctance to cause offence, your trust in cherished stereotypes and your natural ability to be distracted. Many of them are experts at playing mind games.

Mind Games

Playing mind games depends on understanding one or two things about how the human mind works. You can go on courses to learn the art of influencing people. The motives of the attendees at such events may range from a genuine desire to learn how to help people to a decidedly unhelpful urge to use or exploit them. Among the doctors, psychotherapists and teachers, there are likely to be salespeople who want to know how to get you to buy their products, politicians who want to know how to get you to vote for them and possibly the odd sociopath whose motives are far more sinister.

So what is it that they learn on these courses, or discover for themselves by observing people in their everyday lives?

The key to most of it is an understanding of the trance state.

The Trance State

When your attention is fully focused on something inside or outside yourself, as we have already seen, we can be oblivious to whatever else is going on around us. This state of locked attention is the trance state.

We can go into this state automatically or at will, and we do so many times in a typical day. If you are interested in this book, you are probably in the learning trance state right now as you are reading, and that's fine. The point is that you chose to read this and, at any time, you can choose to stop reading and go off and do something else or to stay with it and read the next bit in order to find out some other stuff that you didn't already know.

Voluntary trance states, then, are fine. You can choose to concentrate on watching a game of football or writing a shopping list or listening to a piece of music; it's entirely up to you. It usually works well. Not all trance states, however, are voluntary. Other people can help you into them. This is how hypnosis works.

This present book is not intended to be a manual to teach you how to hypnotise people, so a thorough explanation of how it works and all the different methods of induction is not appropriate here. If you find it fascinating and want to learn more, we can recommend an online webinar by Ivan Tyrell, at the Human Givens College, called 'The Uses and Abuses of Hypnosis'. For now, we'll focus on what you need to know in terms of protecting yourself from those with a tendency to abuse it.

A professional hypnotist, whether the stage version or a clinical hypnotherapist, will, with your permission, carry out a hypnotic induction; in other words, they will help you to reach a relaxed state in which your attention is focused on a particular thing, to the exclusion of everything else.

What we are particularly concerned about here, however, is neither stage hypnosis nor clinical hypnotherapy but the wilful misuse of hypnotic inductions to distract, disorientate and confuse people in order to steal from them, exploit them or cause them physical harm.

As Ivan Tyrell says: "Hypnosis is a form of trespass upon the private mental territory of another. This is territory that you should only enter respectfully if you are invited in and you must be careful to close the gate properly when you leave."

There is nothing respectful about the tactics of the average con artist. An extreme example would be the three (yes three!) double glazing salesmen who turned up on the doorstep of one of our students. Having failed to make a sale, they began to hurl profanities and threats at the student, a gentleman past retirement age who possibly appeared to be a suitable target for intimidation.

They probably knew that loud swearing and threats can put people into a shocked trance state and make them more compliant; it is hard to stay calm and think clearly when someone is shouting in your face.

How wrong they turned out to be! At the point of poking a finger towards the aforementioned gentleman's face, the chief villain in this scenario found himself on the receiving end of a Tai Chi push which resulted in him sitting in the road while his car keys were confiscated, the police were phoned and a crowd of neighbours surrounded all three villains until the police arrived. Our student said afterwards that he had felt quite calm, and had suddenly thought: "I don't have to put up with this; I do Tai Chi."

When people are hurling abuse at you, threatening you or physically abusing you, it's obvious that you need to defend yourself. Some threats are much more subtle or devious than this, however, and we may not know that we've been had until afterwards.

1. The Double Bind

A favourite trick used by salespeople and con artists is the double bind technique in which the 'customer' is presented with a range of options which don't include the option 'none of the above'. For example: "Would you like the red car or the blue car madam?" One might say that political elections work this way! If this subtle use of psychological manipulation seems more to do with self-defence against a perceived threat to your wallet than to your physical safety, remember that one thing can rapidly lead to another. Look for the general principles involved so you can recognise attempts to control and manipulate you.

A favourite scam, which you may already have fallen prey to yourself, is the one where someone comes up to you in the street and says: "You have a kind face. I desperately need to get home. Could you let me have five pounds/bucks for my bus fare or just a few pence/cents if you can spare them?" The implication being that if you think a fiver is too much, you will give them a bit of your loose change rather than appear to be mean and heartless. It's amazing how many people claim to find themselves in this predicament! They can easily be found wandering around the car parks of our cities, or sitting under the ticket machine where you can't avoid them.

They may also use a bit of additional psychology by adding: "That lady over there just gave me (whatever small amount) so all I need is (larger amount but a bit less than the whole amount they 'need')." So you now feel morally obliged to match the other person's generosity rather than look like a skinflint in comparison, and since you have less than the full amount of the original bus fare to donate, you might actually think you're getting a good deal!

Give them money if you want to but do it with your eyes open and don't expect any genuine gratitude and, perhaps more importantly, be alert to the fact that that they may not be alone!

2. The Two-Pronged Hit

Knowing that people can, quite easily, be distracted and put into a trance state, muggers often work in pairs. The first one will usually be a vulnerable-looking person, probably female, who will ask you an innocent sounding question such as: "Could you tell me what time it is, please?" Now at one time, the response of most members of the public would be to look at their watch; these days it's more likely to be a phone. Not only have the villains just confirmed that you have something worth stealing, but your attention is now locked on the task of finding out what time it is.

You are looking at your phone or watch with blinkers on, so you don't notice the accomplice behind you who sticks the point of a knife in your ribs and demands that you remain silent and give them your watch, phone, money or whatever or, worse still, accompany them to some other location.

One lady was abducted in this way from a staircase in a crowded shopping centre and taken to a nearby building where she was assaulted, raped and left for dead. Fortunately, she survived and managed to crawl out onto the street and get help, eventually. She was shocked to find that people avoided her at first because she was naked, dirty and covered in blood. Whether anyone on the staircase in the shopping mall would have rushed to her rescue, had she screamed for help at the start of the attack, is unknown.

Having other people around is not necessarily a guarantee of your safety. When Kitty Genovese was murdered in New York in 1964, the attack lasted for over half an hour and was witnessed by forty people without one of them trying to intervene. There's something about human psychology that makes people reluctant to get involved.

Experiments have shown that the more bystanders there are, the less likely individuals are to take action. When faced with an unusual situation, it may seem to be less of an emergency if other people are remaining calm, and we can justify our failure to help by telling ourselves that we are not personally responsible since nobody else did anything either.

If you're thinking that all this is shocking and that being abducted at knifepoint is probably a very rare occurrence, you need only look up the global statistics on human trafficking and abductions. This is something that is happening all over the world, including in the USA and the UK, and it's not just the odd person here and there, it is millions! There are more slaves in the world today than there were before the abolition of the slave trade, and many of them may have fallen into the hands of gangs as a result of tricks such as these.

Distraction

Not all criminals work with a partner, of course, but they will still use distraction by any means to lock your attention on one thing while they do something you didn't notice, like stealing your wallet or sticking a knife in your ribs. They know that when your attention is distracted and focussed on just one thing, you are in a trance state and you are oblivious to whatever else is going down.

The predator's favourite distraction technique is to engage you in conversation. The order of business is:

Deception - appearing to be harmless, polite and friendly.

Dialogue - getting you talking about something trivial and non-threatening.

Distraction - with your brain focussed on the conversation, your instinctive defences are lowered.

Destruction - a devastating blow that can happen so quickly that most people would not see it coming.

However good you think you are at judging a person's character, and however confident you feel that you can control the situation, your best bet is to avoid getting sucked into any kind of verbal interaction in the first place. If someone you don't know approaches you on the street, just keep walking, whatever they are asking you and whatever sob story they are telling.

If they want to know what time it is; you don't know. If they need directions to that really cool restaurant down the road; you've never heard of it. If they need money; you don't have any. If their poor old grandma just died and they don't have enough money to get to the funeral; tough! Don't get side-tracked into explaining why you can't help them. Whatever their problem is, you are in a hurry and you really can't stop. Walk on. If that sounds cold, it's better than ending up frozen in a mortuary. The general advice to be gleaned from all of this is:

- Stay alert.
- Keep a wide view.
- Trust nobody on the street.
- Be prepared to fight or run.

Dealing with Challenging Behaviour

Not all hazardous people are criminals. There may be ordinary people whose behaviour becomes a potential threat, just because they are angry.

When a person is angry, they are not thinking rationally. This applies to any person and it is a result of how the human mind works, as we saw above.

When we are very emotionally aroused, we allow a very primitive area of our brain, the limbic system, to do our thinking for us. Our rational, thinking mind, the higher cortex, just doesn't get a look in. The only way that we can begin to think rationally again is to calm down and allow the frontal lobes of our brain to come back online.

In other words, there's absolutely no point in arguing with a very angry person, especially if they are drunk or on drugs. Even if they are sober, they are not going to see your point of view, or look for any kind of mutually acceptable solution to whatever it is that's bothering them, until they have calmed down.

Having said that, possibly the worst thing you can say to an angry person is, "Calm down"! The old advice that was given to carers looking after people whose behaviour was often challenging, was to remain seated and speak in a calm voice. At some point, it must have occurred to someone just how patronising and demeaning this sounds to someone who is genuinely frustrated or upset.

So what's the alternative?

Rapport!

Suppose you are working in a complaints office and there is someone standing in front of your desk, shouting at you and using bad language. Maybe you could ignore them, or speak quietly to them in a way that demonstrates your supreme self-control and skills at maintaining meditative tranquillity under difficult circumstances! You can probably think of several good reasons why that strategy sucks.

Maybe you could have them hauled away by the security guards or, if necessary, the police, while pointing to the zero abuse policy notice on the wall. Perhaps, in some cases, this might even be necessary.

Most often, however, this might be an ordinary person in front of you who has an understandable grievance and needs a really good listening to, in which case you could try the following.

1. Mirror the person's body language. If possible, stand up so that your face is level with theirs.

2. Listen to what they are saying and summarise the main points they are making, as you understand them. If you don't understand, ask them for more clarification and then repeat what you heard, raising your voice a little so that it almost matches theirs. "Are you telling me that you've been charged twice for the same item and you couldn't get through to our helpline? No wonder you're concerned! Anyone would be. Shall we sit down and see if we can find out what's been going on so that we can sort it out for you."

3. Only then sit down, lower your voice as you continue the conversation, have a look at the records and do what you can

to help the person, out of genuine concern for their needs. (They will know if you really couldn't give a damn.)

It is amazing how quickly a person can calm down when you respond in this way. What they now know is that someone is finally listening to them; somebody actually understands their problem and is trying to help them. You have 'normalised' their situation so they no longer feel alone in their frustration. Don't be surprised if tears well up in their eyes as the stress they have been bottling up inside them bubbles to the surface. They now see themselves, and you, as 'concerned', rather than angry, and they are ready to sit down so that you can both work together to solve the problem.

Even if you can't offer any practical help, they still know that you appreciate how difficult that must be for them and they are less likely to blame you personally for the situation. Perhaps you can then offer advice on where to go for help or how to register a formal complaint about the system. Either way, you have protected yourself, and perhaps others around you, from further verbal, and possibly physical, abuse while also allowing the person an opportunity to gain better access to their own rational mind as they work out how to get through the crisis.

You may be asking yourself: 'How is this relevant to a book about Tai Chi?' Or maybe you can see a bit of Yin and Yang creeping in here. Perhaps a little Wu Wei, going with the flow, rather than rising to the bait, getting into a shouting match and pouring oil onto the flames. Tai Chi is all about avoiding and resolving conflict wherever possible.

Notice that you are mirroring a person's aroused state, not becoming over-emotional yourself. Allowing yourself to become angry leads to a conflict situation in which we now have two illogical people, without a rational thought between them, trying to use the emotional, primitive parts of their brains to solve a tricky problem!

We hope you never find yourself in a situation where physical self-defence is necessary. This has been quite a long chapter because our main aim is to help you to be alert, be aware, evaluate the situation and avoid any kind of violent conflict, if at all possible.

We will now move on to Step 7, in which we will offer some suggestions on how to be prepared for physical conflict if it were ever to become unavoidable, all else having failed to avert it, and what to do to help to increase the odds of your survival.

Step 7

Be Prepared

'The opportunity to flee a confrontation is the first choice. Without a heightened state of awareness the individual will not see a problem arise and will be taken by surprise. This must not be allowed to happen – stay 'switched on'.'

The British Combat Association

By now, you will have realised that the best way to protect yourself is to avoid getting into difficult situations in the first place. That might not always be possible but you can increase your chances of staying out of trouble by being aware of the kinds of tactics criminals use and by staying alert at all times.

Being aware and alert is not the same as being paranoid. If you are driving a car, you don't have to be in a state of perpetual anxiety to wear a seat belt and keep a watchful eye out for other road users: you are just aware of potential risks and taking sensible precautions.

If you are walking down the street, you don't need to be tense, anxious and hyper-vigilant; in fact that kind of mental state shows up as fear to anyone watching you and, as we saw in the section on self-awareness, predators are more likely to target you if you behave in that way.

Being alert just means that you are fully present in the moment, not caught up in thoughts about the past or the future. Call it mindfulness if you like. Your attention is wide open in all directions. As well as helping you to avoid difficult situations, being aware and alert is also the best state to be in if you were ever to find yourself, unavoidably, in such a situation.

A Wider View

Even without the deliberate distractions provided by villains on the street, most of us tend to do a pretty good job of distracting ourselves most of the time, not just with our electronic gadgets or other external objects but also with the stuff that goes on inside our own heads.

It's possible to be pretty much wrapped up in our own thoughts from the moment we wake up until we fall asleep at night. Not only does that use up a lot of mental and emotional energy; it also puts us into an almost perpetual trance state in which we are oblivious to what is going on around us. If we are busy going over what someone said to us this morning and rehearsing what we will say to them later today, we are not fully aware of what is happening right here and now, and that makes us vulnerable.

The antidote to a trance state is to bring yourself into the present and open up your awareness in all directions. Sounds easy but, like any other skill, it can take a bit of practice if you are not used to it.

Have a go at this exercise right now:

1. Open up your peripheral vision. While still looking at the page in front of you, be aware of what you can see to either side on the edges of your visual field.
2. Open up your hearing, including the furthest, faintest sounds from all directions.

Practice this skill as often as you can remember to do it. Let it become a habit.

Try it when you are practicing a Tai Chi sequence, or pushing hands with a partner, or sitting in a garden or walking down the street. You can do it in a busy office or a shopping mall; you can do it while you're dancing or eating your lunch. Just be there, be present and be aware.

It may not seem like much but this simple shift in perspective has instantly switched you from 'sleep' mode to 'alert' mode. This has three immediate effects:

- You are now more likely to notice any potential threats.

- Your body language will now give out signals that you are switched on so it's best not to mess with you.

- You also get to notice some of the pleasant things in life that you might otherwise have missed.

Living 'mindfully' isn't all about self-protection, it's also about appreciating what's here and now: hearing what a small child is trying to say to you, noticing the taste of your food and taking time to enjoy the fragrance of honeysuckle on the evening air.

Generally though, if you are out and about, you can ramp your level of awareness up and down as necessary, using the following 'Traffic Light' system.

Traffic Lights

The following is based on the UK traffic signalling system and may be different if you live in another country. The colours you use don't matter as long as they work for you and you have a three stage preparation in mind, such as:

Green for Go on as Normal

Once you develop the habit of paying attention, you will be walking down the street alert and prepared and, while everything is normal, you have green for go: you are just going about your business as usual.

Yellow Alert for Caution

If you notice something unusual that could potentially turn into a risk situation, you move to code amber or yellow alert. You are more cautious and looking for ways of avoiding any unpleasantness. This might not even be a risk you can see and identify. It could just be an instinct that something is not quite right. Prepare to get out of there if you need to. Cross the street to avoid that group of guys on the corner or say "no thanks" to the person offering to help you to carry your stuff into your room.

Red Alert for Emergency Action

If the suspicious-looking character approaching you just walks right on by, you can move back down to code green, but if the 'threat' turns out to be real, you go to code red – take emergency action. If you can run, get out of there as fast as you can. If you can't run, prepare to fight, if necessary.

If you can't remember the various colours of the traffic light system, don't worry about it, just stay alert and aware and listen to your instincts if there is anything unusual going on around you. You might feel perfectly at ease as you walk around your local supermarket but if you see a suspicious looking package, or if someone walks in wearing a balaclava or if that lady next to you seems to be unnaturally close to you, move out of the way first and ask questions later.

Listen to your 'sixth sense'!

If your intuition is telling you that something isn't right, pay attention. A student of ours was walking home from a bus stop when she felt a 'creepy' sensation in the back of her neck and instinctively turned around and lashed out with her bag, which struck the face of the guy behind her who was preparing to grab her by the hair! Although she had a black belt in Karate, she knew better than to stick around and test her best moves on this low-life, so she ran home using the adrenalin boost to give her wings!

Avoid conflict in any way you can

Do whatever you can to talk your way out of trouble. Be nice to people, but not too nice (remember the gazelle in the last chapter).

People have actually been maimed or killed by road users who took exception to their lack of courtesy, even over something as seemingly trivial as not saying thank you when someone stopped to let them go first.

On the other hand, never wind down your window to speak to an irate motorist. Road rage is a thing! One lady had her nose bitten off by a guy who was annoyed because she spent too long hesitating at a road junction!

In general, though, a little courtesy can often go a long way. We had a student who had, before taking up Tai Chi, spent many years in the military and confessed that he had a very short fuse and was known for his ability to handle himself. He had a habit of using his fists at the slightest provocation and it was therefore with some degree of surprise that he told us of an incident that occurred after he had been practicing Tai Chi for a while.

He had been driving his van down a narrow street on a wet day and his wheel had passed through a large puddle and soaked a nearby pedestrian: a big guy who was not particularly pleased by this experience, as evidenced by the subsequent stream of abuse he hurled after the van. Now, at one time, our student told us, he would have immediately risen to the challenge and a fist fight might have ensued. But strangely, he felt inwardly calm – a phenomenon he attributed to the Tai Chi. He parked the van and got out saying: 'Sorry mate. Didn't see that puddle. You OK?' He was not only surprised by his own response to the situation but also amazed to see the effect it had on the wet pedestrian, whose anger seemed to evaporate away. After a short conversation, both men were on the best of terms and a potential conflict had been avoided.

Our student said that this experience had changed his life. He felt like a new man, with a new perspective on the world.

As we have said many times:

Self-protection, by awareness and avoidance of trouble, is always the first choice.

Self-defence, on the other hand, is a last-ditch resort. It's what you do when everything else - all the alertness, awareness and avoidance strategies – has not worked and you are face to face with someone who poses an immediate threat.

So far we have focussed, in great detail, on how to avoid trouble if you can. From now on we will look very closely at what to do if you have no alternative but to fight.

Recognise the Signs

Other than a complete surprise attack from behind, it is very rare for a physical attack to occur without warning. Before a physical attack occurs, there will be warning signs and you can learn to notice and identify them.

Whatever a person may be saying to you, their body language and physical state will tell you much more about their real intentions. Aggressors usually give out lots of non-verbal clues prior to an attack.

Often known as 'ritualised combat', warning signs of a possible attack may progress to danger signs indicative of an imminent attack.

Warning signs

- *Prolonged eye contact* – a sign of dominance and aggression which is sometimes a sign of scared bullies who don't want to fight and so just try to intimidate you instead. At other times, however, staring is a sign that someone really wants to harm you.

- *Facial colour darkens* when people are embarrassed. It's very dangerous to embarrass people - they resent it.

- *Standing tall* - head back and chin lifted, chest out - is a macho thing; intimidation by looking big and 'hard'. Sticking out their jaw can be a sign that someone is beginning to feel aggressive.

- *Large movements, arms wide* - may be body language for "I'll fight you!"

- *Rapid breathing* – a sign that adrenalin is kicking in, for whatever reason. Fear and anger are equally dangerous because both can lead to aggression.

All of the above tell you that an attack is possible. The following tell you that an attack is actually about to happen:

Danger signs

- *Eye flicking* – eyes darting around, perhaps checking for witnesses, planning escape routes and sizing up their target.

- *Fist clenching* ready to punch you.

- *Face pales.* This is beyond the redness of mere anger. It is a sign that they are ramped up with adrenalin and ready to come at you.

- *Lips tighten over teeth* – Biting happens so be aware of it.

- *Eyebrows drop* to protect the eyes.

- *Head drops forward* to protect the throat

- *Shoulders tense* like a Rottweiler with hackles raised.

- *Hands raise above waist* ready to attack you *OR hands in pockets*. They may have a knife or a gun. If someone approaches you with their hands in their pockets, stay well, back, out of their way. People have been stabbed multiple times within seconds as someone walked past them with a concealed weapon. A knife could also be hidden in a bag such as fast-food packaging.

- *The aggressor breaks eye contact* and looks at their intended target.

- *Stance changes from square to side on.* In some cases, especially when the attacker is smaller than you, they may look away before hitting you. This can be a type of deception where they say they don't want any trouble and pretend they are about to walk away. They back off and turn their body slightly to the side but then they suddenly turn towards you again and throw a fist at you, using the circular momentum to generate more force.

- If the attacker is an experienced fighter, *their body may lower* just before they attack

Close Quarter Strategies

In a real fight, you don't get time to scroll through a list of strategies, moves and counter-moves or evaluate the potential benefits of eighty-five types of jin. A lot of what takes place will happen very quickly and spontaneously, on an unconscious level, and The Fight, Flight or Freeze Response will be involved, hitting you with an adrenalin dump early on.

Martial arts training is designed to programme your unconscious responses so that, like the old lady who punched the guy in the gut in the opening paragraph of this book, your body does something spontaneous and helpful before you even have time to think about it and therefore possibly even before the adrenalin hits you.

Don't be surprised however if the shock of the situation turns your legs to jelly and causes you to freeze momentarily. That just means you are human. You can still get through this and a bit of prior knowledge of what to expect can help you to unfreeze yourself and do something useful.

Most of this book has been about how to train your Tai Chi skills in readiness for such a situation. Here are a few essential rules of real combat.

- *SWEAR!* Abusive language is a part of real-life combat. Accept it, expect it, use it if necessary and don't let it phase you.

- *BACK OFF!* Don't try to handle the situation by yourself if you can get away and get help.

- *DON'T WAIT FOR THEM TO STRIKE YOU!*

If there is no possibility of getting away:

- *Control the pre-fight* – Be assertive rather than meek and compliant (which is what they want) or hostile and aggressive (which can escalate the situation).

- *Control the space* – control the distance between yourself and the attacker. Step back or to the side, if possible.

- *Use a 'fence' or guard* - keep your hands between yourself and your attacker. It takes too long to raise your arms from your sides if someone is about to hit you. Keep your hands at chest height in what appears to be a placatory gesture but which allows you to control the space and intercept any incoming attack. This is where the Tai Chi posture Play Guitar (strum the lute/pippa) is useful but don't make it look like a martial arts pose, which could be seen as a challenge to fight you. Keep it subtle and with palms towards the attacker.

- *Try to use verbal dissuasion.* If possible, give them a way to back off without losing face. Sometimes, people go ahead with an attack because they see no alternative. One of us once intercepted a menacing approach by a huge mountain of a guy with the comment: "Wow! Awesome muscles, mate! You must have worked hard to get those!" At which point aggression gave way to mutual back-slapping and a shared round of drinks! Rapport can still be established even at this late stage, as long you provide what Geoff Thompson calls a "loophole" that allows the situation to go a different way without making anyone look bad.

- *If they move forward, PUSH THEM BACK!* A double palm strike to the chest can cause a massive adrenaline dump in your attacker, similar to fear, and it might just make them hesitate or even back off.

- *Back this up with a verbal shout*: "GET BACK! GET THE F*** BACK!"

- *Use a pre-emptive strike – HIT THEM FIRST!* If they try to get past your guard, they have made the first move and you have every right to finish the fight right there, so…

- *Use your TOOLS* (see below for a list) and…

- *FINISH THE FIGHT IN THREE SECONDS* (if you can) *or RUN AWAY* (if you can)

- If your first strike misses its target, *KEEP AT THEM* until you knock them out or get an opportunity to escape. You can act like a crazy person if you want to. The ability to fight is programmed into you by millions of years of evolution and only recently suppressed in our civilised society. Some drug users and maniacs can't be held down by half a dozen police men because their behaviour is uninhibited and they are fuelled by their adrenalin. Lose your inhibitions and tap into the vast reserves of adrenalin you will undoubtedly have at your disposal. Don't let it cripple you, use it!

If you have ever trained in a Tai Chi technique called 'a thousand hands guan yin', which is basically walking towards your opponent firing rapid palm strikes or punches over and over like a maniac, then this might be a good time to do that.

"Avoid, escape, loophole, posture and, if you have to be physical, be first and be ferocious." - Geoff Thompson.

The above advice applies equally to men and women but it tends to conjure up an image of a man preparing to punch another man. Of course, the attack might not be a punch and, if you are female, the objective of a male attacker might be to grab your arms, throat or hair, back you against a wall or knock you to the floor. A female attacker might be trying to kick you, scratch you or slap you, though. In reality, anything is possible, whatever your gender or that of your attacker.

The above also assumes that the attacker is in front of you, when in fact many attacks occur from behind or while walking past very quickly perhaps with a knife concealed in a pocket or a fast food bag, and the victim never sees it coming.

Awareness is paramount! Be alert, trust your instincts and get away if you can.

Is this Tai Chi?

In this chapter, we talk a lot about pre-emptive strikes. You may be wondering: does all this talk about pre-emptive strikes contradict our Tai Chi training? Let's think about that.

According to the Tai Chi classics, there is a difference between Tai Chi and other martial arts. In most martial arts, the victory goes to the strongest and the fastest and the idea is to get the first blow in before the opponent has a chance to retaliate.

In Tai Chi, on the other hand, we are taught that even a small, weak or elderly person can defeat a big, fit bloke by letting them make the first move and then doing the whole intercept, stick, deflect thing, thereby 'using four ounces to overcome a thousand pounds'.

Well yes but that doesn't mean that you should stand there and take one on the jaw, just to see what your opponent has got! That one punch could be the last thing you see of this world! A better sentence to recall from the Tai Chi classics is 'my opponent moves a little; I move first'.

You move first because, internally, you are already moving. Your hands are already raised and controlling the space, and the explosion of your force can hit them before they have had time to launch their attack. So yes, you move first with your pre-emptive strike, not necessarily in response to their incoming fist but in response to their *intention* to hit you

Wu Yuxian described three timings in martial arts. In modern terms, these are referred to as 'before, during and after' but the old masters talked about them as energies.

- *Striking the contained energy* means hitting them at the moment of intent, as they may be coming into range but have not yet primed themselves ready to hit you.

- *Striking the incoming energy* means that they have already launched their attack and you are intercepting, parrying and simultaneously striking, as we have described in detail in the section on jin.

- *Striking the retreating energy* is when you have evaded their attack and they withdraw and you follow them during their retreat to strike them, pin them, knock them over or do whatever else is necessary.

Cheng Man Ching described a technique called 'Ti Fang' which means 'lifting and moving'. This involves enticing an opponent to over-reach with a strike and then evading the incoming blow, allowing you to seize the attacker's arm, lock it up and use it to lift the person and set them down somewhere else. This seemingly bizarre technique can be surprisingly effective, as the opponent is over-committed and their arm is locked out and vulnerable.

From the legendary tale of the fight between a snake and a crane, we learn that jumping backwards like the crane is a good move if you have the legs for it! If you have nowhere to escape to, then becoming the snake is recommended. Just remember that a snake not only wriggles and writhes to escape capture, it also strikes and spits poison!

Tai Chi on the Street

Most of this book has been about how Tai Chi can allow you to develop the unconscious skills that could improve your chances of dealing with various types of attempted assault if you are aware enough and lucky enough to see it coming but don't have the option of getting away from your attacker without some kind of physical contact taking place.

Among the most useful fighting skills that Tai Chi can teach you are:

- How to stay on your feet and avoid being taken to the ground (by sinking and rooting),

- How to wriggle out of an opponent's attempted grasp like a snake and

- How to hit someone with enough explosive force to knock them out and give you an opportunity to escape.

When it comes to the applications of Tai Chi movements, do be aware that many of the ones you may have seen on YouTube can seem very impressive when performed against a cooperative partner but they would be very unlikely to be useful in a real violent confrontation. Throughout this book, we have attempted to focus on principles and strategies that could actually help to save you from harm.

Although we have focussed mainly on empty-hand techniques, remember that in a real fight there are no rules and you need to use any weapons available to you, including the various parts of your body and anything in the immediate area that you can lay your hands on or get between yourself and your attacker.

Tools

Whether you are armed or unarmed, you still have weapons. As you will see in a moment, practically every part of your body is a potential weapon. If there are additional tools around you, so much the better. In a serious conflict, you may need to use any weapon available.

You might have trained with swords and a spear but it is unlikely that you would have one to hand in a real fight on the street unless you're carrying one illegally or on your way to or from class with your sword bag over your shoulder.

That doesn't mean that your weapons training was wasted, however. You have 'transferable skills' that may help you to use any kind of stick effectively for self-protection. Depending on where you are, you may be able to grab a snooker cue, sweeping brush, rake, walking stick, umbrella, rolled-up newspaper/magazine or washing line prop.

At closer range, an effective weapon might be a comb, pen, pencil, keys, nail file, bottle, hair brush or a cup of coffee, any type of aerosol spray, perfume, household cleaning fluid, fire extinguisher or pressure hose. Even a credit card thrust into the attacker's face or eye might buy you a few seconds in which to escape.

Even if you are completely unarmed, remember that you still have a whole arsenal of weapons! These are:

- Hands (palms, fingers, thumbs, fingernails, fists)

- Arms (wrists, forearms, elbows, upper arms, shoulders)

- Legs (Toes, feet, heels, shins, knees, thighs, hips)

- Head

- Teeth

- Chest

- Back

And remember that your voice is a weapon. Use abusive language - loudly!

Shout "GET F***ING BACK!"

If you hit them, hit them hard and shout in their face. The 'hwa' breath that engages the dantien and releases the full force of your internal power can become a mighty: "HWAAAA!"

When somebody roars like a maniac in your face, it tends to startle you a bit. It can even make you freeze momentarily or put you into a trance state. If you can do that to your attacker, it might just buy you a precious second or two in which to escape or follow through with the move that knocks them out cold. At the very least, it might attract the attention of other people. Whether or not any onlookers decide to come to your aid, your attacker might be uncomfortable with an audience and decide it's not worth the risk.

So attract as much attention as you can. Shout, scream; use an alarm if you have one. If someone tries to get you into a car, shout: "I don't know you!" so that bystanders don't think this is a family dispute, which might make them less likely to 'get involved'. You can also shout "Someone please help me! Call the police!" Even if nobody dares to come to your rescue, they might do the popular thing these days: get out their mobile phone and take pictures. Your attacker might just have second thoughts about having a video of his actions shown in court or going viral on YouTube!

Very recently, another female student of ours was walking through a Christmas market when a man bumped into her. She continued on her way but felt that someone was behind her and she turned to find the man's hand inside her bag. Before he had a chance to steal anything she pointed at him, shouting "YOU'RE A THIEF! GET BACK! GET YOUR HAND OUT OF MY BAG!" People around were now watching and the man pulled his hood around his face and escaped into the crowd without managing to take anything from the bag. Your voice is a weapon. Use it!

If you can't run away, then make use of anything that you can get between yourself and your attacker, particularly if they have a knife.

Chairs, tables and desks can create a barrier. A small chair can be picked up and used as a weapon.

There might be things that you can throw: soil, stones, clocks, pans, crockery, a book, a coat, a computer or ornaments - basically anything that you can lift and that isn't nailed down! If you are wearing high heeled shoes, take them off and throw them. You can run faster without them anyway.

One of us once found herself on a grassy hillside in front of six stampeding rhinos. Unarmed and with nothing to hide behind, had she tried to run away, she would have been swiftly overtaken, so she ran towards them shouting and throwing handfuls of grass! Fortunately for her, rhinos are quite short-sighted and her intimidating behaviour was scary enough to make them turn around and run back up the hill.

We are not suggesting that you should sign up for a course in self-defence against rampant wildlife, unless you happen to be working as a Game Warden, as in this case, but there's a principle here: Having things thrown at you by a crazy person is not a comfortable experience for most people. We already know from psychological research that predators tend to prefer targets who are quiet and submissive so that they can do what they do without injury to themselves and without being caught.

Shortly after one of us had faced down six rampant rhinos, elsewhere in the world, the other, with a friend, found themselves being pursued by half a dozen equally hostile and hardly more intellectually evolved, humans. During the process of legging it, the thought suddenly occurred: "Why are we running?" At which point, they stopped and turned round. This strategy, while not necessarily recommended in every situation, threw the chasing pack into confusion. It seems that they had been enjoying the thrill of the chase and had not anticipated the possibility of engaging in actual combat or being subjected to return fire of verbal threats and insults. The battle was over very quickly as they thought better of it and went home.

Lots of luck involved? Perhaps, but we do know that many would-be assailants are likely to be seeking domination and control of a weaker person. They want you to be scared and back away and may think twice if you do the opposite. The elderly student who punched her mugger in the gut was quite frail and her assailant could easily have overpowered her. What gave her the advantage was the element of surprise - big guys don't expect to be punched by old ladies - and the fact that he now had an audience: an entire shopping mall full of witnesses! Like the guy at the Christmas market mentioned earlier: he had planned to grab her bag quietly, before anyone noticed. Instead, he found himself the star of a public performance and he had no choice but to get out of there as fast as possible.

Shouting and throwing things at someone, then, may attract attention and give your assailant second thoughts, unless they happen to be pointing a gun at you, in which case it's probably best to give them your wallet, your phone or whatever else they are asking for. Staying alive tends to be generally preferable to any last moment acts of heroism.

Training with Weapons

The traditional weapons used in Tai Chi Chuan include the broadsword (Dao), the straight sword (Jian), the long spear and the staff.

Even blunt or wooden practice swords are actually quite dangerous and must be carried discreetly to and from classes. You might wonder,

178

then, why anyone might want to train in the use of weapons that can't be used in any practical self-protection situation.

There are several reasons why we believe that training with weapons is an important aspect of Tai Chi Chuan. Quite apart from the aesthetic beauty of a Tai Chi weapons sequence practiced as an art form, the weight of it can strengthen muscles, particularly in your arms, and contribute to your general health and fitness. From a self-protection viewpoint, it allows you to develop skills that translate to any other similar object that might be available in a fight.

Training with swords develops skills that would help you to use something of a similar size to defend yourself with, such as a walking stick or umbrella. However, it should also give you a healthy respect for knives of any length. There is no safe way to disarm an attacker who is threatening you with a knife, whatever you might read about such methods or see demonstrated on videos, and whatever techniques you may use in class to 'defang the snake' by striking the hand or wrist of a cooperative fellow student. Getting yourself out of there or getting a barrier such as a table, chair, coat or car between yourself and your assailant is infinitely preferable to any ideas you might have of taking the weapon from him or her.

Spear training allows you to get used to wielding a long stick, such as a clothes prop, and the shaking of a spear or rattan cane can help you to develop the ability to use your body to generate waves of energy or fa jin.

Training with sticks of varying lengths can give you some very practical skills that would help you to make use of anything to hand in a crisis, from a garden rake or sweeping brush to a rolled up magazine or newspaper.

With any weapons sequence, all the general Tai Chi principles are still required, from stable postures, sinking and rooting to fluidity of movement and correct breathing, and the types of jin we have explored still apply, from intercepting and sticking to neutralising and issuing. The result of training should be that the weapon becomes an extension of your arm and you are able to send your 'energy' along it in the same way that you would send it into your hands and fingers in a hand form.

However, the intention should be to defend yourself rather than to look for ways to attack. Once you launch your attack, you leave areas of your body exposed to an opponent's counter-attack. If you lunge with a sword, for example, you need to be absolutely sure that your opponent has been incapacitated to the point where it is not possible for them to take advantage of your over-committed stance, which would take too much time for you to recover from.

Your weapon should form a protective shield between yourself and your opponent.

Keep your attention wide and fluid rather than allowing your gaze to become locked on the opponent's weapon so you don't miss the other guy with a broken bottle who is sneaking up behind you.

Get out of there as fast as you can.

Your Legal Right to Use Force

The following section describes your legal rights if you are living in the UK. If you live elsewhere, you will need to find out the local and national laws relating to self-protection in your state or country and keep abreast of any changes.

Human Rights Act 1998 (Article 2)

The use of force must be:

- REASONABLE under all the circumstances,

- PROPORTIONAL to the seriousness of the crime,

- ABSOLUTELY NECESSARY under the circumstances,

- HAVE LEGAL AUTHORITY under established legislation.

The Criminal Law Act 1967 (Section 3)

Any person may use 'such force as is reasonable in the prevention of crime, or in the effecting or assisting in the lawful arrest of offenders or suspected offenders or persons unlawfully at large. (This force) must not be disproportionate to the mischief to be averted.'

For example, citizens can arrest someone for theft, damage or assault, but not for parking outside their house! If an arrest is justified, be careful. People have been killed while trying to arrest thieves stealing their cars!

The law has since been further clarified by:

Section 76 of the Criminal Justice and Immigration Act 2008

This goes into great detail about the degree of force that is reasonable, considering the circumstances, as seen by the person defending themselves. Householders confronting an intruder in their own home can use force that is 'disproportionate' but not 'grossly disproportionate'. In a court of law, the individual circumstances of the householder will be considered, along with 'the threat (real or perceived) posed by the offender'.

Section 76(7) states that: 'evidence of a person's having only done what the person honestly and instinctively thought was necessary for a legitimate purpose constitutes strong evidence that only reasonable action was taken by that person for that purpose.'

It is acknowledged that 'a person acting for a legitimate purpose may not be able to weigh to a nicety the exact measure of any necessary action'.

So don't let fear of an assault charge prevent you from doing whatever you believe is necessary to protect yourself and your family but don't go overboard and become vindictive.

For example, when two of our elderly students restrained an intruder by sitting on him until the police arrived, they were using reasonable force in the circumstances. Had he posed a greater threat, they might have needed to knock him out or to do whatever they considered to be necessary for their survival. However, if they had decided to beat him up or subject him to some kind of sadistic torture while he lay there passively, in order to 'teach him a lesson', that would clearly have been 'grossly disproportionate'.

Common Law

'A person has a right to defend themselves from attack, to act in the defence of others, to arrest offenders and, if necessary, to use force on another in so doing. If no more force is used than is reasonable to repel the attack, such force is not unlawful and no crime is committed. Circumstances may justify a pre-emptive strike.'

When asked by the police if you used reasonable force, your answer will be key evidence. If you say "Well I don't know, maybe I could have used a bit less..." this may provide grounds for a case against you. For example, an elderly female student of ours was charged with assault for pushing over a man in his twenties who had burgled her house and was attempting to hit her over the head with a hammer, though later the case was dismissed.

Pre-emptive Strikes

According to the website of the Crown Prosecution Service: 'There is no rule in law to say that a person must wait to be struck first before they may defend themselves.'

If you let them hit you, that may be your very last action in this lifetime! If you believe that someone is a threat, don't be afraid to hit them first.

How to use a pre-emptive strike to finish the fight in seconds.

You may have seen top fighters go ten rounds with an opponent. You may even have survived several gruelling bouts of push hands in a competition. On the street, however, things tend to happen very fast and the whole thing is usually over in seconds, before you even have time to think about it.

The attacker is in his or her own arena of choice and may have done this kind of thing before many times. There are no rules and it is unlikely that anyone will step in to help you. There is no possibility of any kind of gentlemanly conduct. The fight needs to be ended then and there and you need to do it first, before they do. So where and how do you hit them?

Targets

The Eyes

If an attacker, can't see you they have less chance of hurting you. You will no doubt have seen people in movies throwing sand in an opponent's face. Spraying them with mace or hairspray can be equally effective, but so can deliberately striking them in the eyes with your fingers. Even poking your finger deeply into one eye can cause both eyes to close and give you time to escape. You can also use a sideways flick with the fingers rather than a poking action. Even if you miss, or if your attacker is wearing glasses, going for the eyes can cause them to flinch, allowing you an instant of time in which to deliver a punch or palm strike to their jaw.

The Jaw

Striking anywhere along the jawbone, from the chin to the ear, can potentially send a shockwave through the head and shake the brain, causing concussion and unconsciousness.

The Neck

A strike to the front of the throat can damage the windpipe (oesophagus) but there is a bony protrusion that can also damage your fist. A little to the left or right of that, between the Adams apple and the ear, the tissues are softer and there are nerves and blood vessels that supply the brain. A blow in this area can temporarily cut off the supply of blood to the brain, again leading to unconsciousness.

Other Targets

All of the above depends on having clear access to your attacker's head and neck. If they are wearing a helmet or if they are much taller than you and their arms are in the way, you may need to find a lower target, even if only to get them to lower their arms so that you can get a clear shot at their jaw.

The Liver

People have been brought down by a powerful blow beneath the ribs on the right side of their body. Notice that, if you are right handed, their liver is on the opposite side to your strong fist, so it can be difficult to pull this off unless you are good at delivering a blow with your left hand or if they have turned that side towards you.

A well placed elbow strike to this area, however, might be easier to achieve. Elbow strikes can also be very effective if your opponent is beside or behind you. So don't become over reliant on your hands; remember all the other tools available.

The Heart and the Solar Plexus

Striking someone in the chest along their centre line can cause heart irregularities, and striking upwards in the mid area below their ribs can knock the wind out of them in much the same way as the Heimlich manoeuvre in First Aid.

The Groin

This is not normally a preferred target as it only works with male attackers. Understandably, most men will have developed unconscious reflexes to protect this vulnerable region.

Having said that, a kick, punch, finger jab or grab and pull in this area can be very effective if you are very quick and they don't see it coming.

An elderly female student of ours was leaving a class at a health club and was confronted by a man as she went to her car one afternoon. Her immediate instinct was to kick him very hard in the groin, which is not normally a recommended strategy but in her case it worked well as his cry of agony and doubled-up appearance attracted the attention of the security guard and other people in the car park and the man was apprehended.

The Knee and the Shin

Tai Chi kicks, as you know, are normally aimed very low, and with good reason. If you are young, fit and have trained for many years in kick boxing or a similar sport, you may be so adept at delivering spinning back kicks that you can pull one off in a crisis situation, with adrenalin pumping in your veins, and hit your target square on the jaw and land back on your feet again with no problem at all.

For most normal people, this tactic is likely to get you injured, killed or at the very least, laying on your back with your opponent on top of you.

Kicking hard with a toe or a heel to a target no more than a couple of feet above the ground is within the capabilities of most people, even elderly people and children.

A kick to the shin can be very painful. A kick to the knee can be debilitating and prevent your attacker from coming after you as you run away.

Tip! Only use a toe kick if you are wearing strong shoes, otherwise you will end up being the one who is left hobbling! If you have bare feet or you are wearing slippers, flip-flops or soft shoes, kick with your heel.

Percussive Strikes versus Tai Chi Strikes

Now here's where there might be some controversy between Tai Chi practitioners and other martial artists.

Suppose you have a clear shot at your opponent's face.

Do you go for the eyes, the jaw or the throat? Do you use a finger jab or Dian Xue/Dim Mak point strike, or a fist or a palm strike? If you use a fist, do you use a percussive jab, a hook, a cross or a Tai Chi 'one-inch punch'?

In fact we probably shouldn't be asking such questions because over-thinking can lead to indecision over what to do, and that can cause you to hesitate and give an advantage to your attacker. The central message of this book is to train your responses to the point where they will kick in spontaneously without you having to think about it.

However, now that we have mentioned it, it's probably worth examining these questions more closely at this stage, while you are safely here reading this book, so that you can decide which skills to train.

Percussive strikes

Let's start by looking at the conventional wisdom of percussive strikes. There are excellent books available on the subject and excellent teachers around who will train you in how to deliver a hook, a jab, a cross and various combinations. Some of the best teachers have spent long years working as doormen or security guards and the techniques they train are well tried and tested in real life situations on the street.

What we're saying here is that everything is useful if it works and it saves your life. So when we talk about Tai Chi strikes and punches we're not undervaluing the great wealth of combat experience gained by other fighters throughout history, we're just exploring another way of doing things. In the end we should find a balance between hard and soft techniques and be able to use either or both if we need to.

At the very least, we should be aware of them so that we are ready to deal with them if an attacker uses them against us.

The Jab and the Back-fist.

These punches are strong and may be so fast that you don't see them coming, yet they are unlikely to knock out an attacker. That doesn't mean they are not useful, however. They can give the attacker a bloody nose or get them to flinch, which can buy you time to deliver a more devastating blow. A slap to the face can have the same effect.

The Cross and the Hook Punch

A cross or hook is more likely to be the blow that finishes the fight, if it hits an appropriate target such as the jaw line. The idea is to cause the attacker's head to jerk back violently, which shakes the brain inside the skull, potentially causing unconsciousness and giving you time to run away.

In other words, your best bet is to cause a shock wave to travel through your assailant's head!

Now, as a Tai Chi practitioner, you should know all about generating shock waves!

Tai Chi Strikes and Punches

A blow delivered on target with fa jin is likely to cause a shock wave through the opponent, whatever part of the body it is aimed at.

Fa jin can be generated from your whole body through any part of you that is in contact with your adversary.

Potentially, this changes the game because it means that you don't have to waste time withdrawing an arm and leaving yourself vulnerable in order to generate enough momentum to deliver a good cross or hook punch.

If your hand is already close to your opponent's face, such as after a failed strike to the eyes, you can use it to follow through with a cannon fist or palm strike to the jaw with that same hand.

The Eyes then Jaw combination

In more conventional fighting, where you are relying on percussive strikes alone, a good strategy might be to target the eyes with your weak hand (or lead hand) so that, if you don't succeed, you can then follow through with your strong hand to deliver a knockout punch to the jaw.

That's a good strategy that might work, and indeed it has worked out there in the real world, but there are a couple of things to consider here.

Your weak hand is unlikely to hit the target as it goes for the eyes, unless you have an exceptional level of skill and accuracy. That doesn't mean you shouldn't do it though, as anything going towards a person's eyes is likely to cause them to at least blink or flinch, giving you time to hit them with your strong hand, or at least that's the theory.

What we have found in practice is that the opponent immediately throws up their arms to protect their face and then retaliates while you look for other things to do now that the jaw line is no longer available as your strong hand's intended target.

It would probably have been better to have hit the jaw first without bothering about the eyes.

Even if they don't fling their arms upwards, it takes time for a percussive strike to reach its target; time in which your opponent can cover up and counter or knock you over or kick you, once they have sensed what you are about to do.

A pre-emptive strike, then, is best delivered out of the blue, before an attacker is aware that it is happening.

Does that mean don't go for the eyes at all? Actually no: it just means that the left, right combination is not something we would consider to be advisable but, as you know, there is an alternative.

As a Tai Chi practitioner, it might be possible to deliver both strikes with the same hand.

This gives you three advantages:

1. You save time by not having to change hands or even having to withdraw your arm between strikes.

2. If you strike to the eyes with your strong hand, you are more likely to hit the target precisely and, even if not, your strong hand is already there in your attacker's face, ready to send a shockwave through the jaw without wasting time by withdrawing your arm to launch a percussive strike.

3. Your weaker hand can be otherwise occupied in controlling your attacker's arms while this is going on.

We have previously discussed the wrapping motion, both arms circling in the same direction, one after the other. If you practice this with a partner, many times, you will eventually train an automatic response that can be very fast and very effective.

As to eyes or jaw, that's up to you but if you go for the eyes, follow through with a fist or palm strike to the jaw anyway rather than pause first to see if it worked. There's a lot of truth in the saying: 'He (or indeed she) who hesitates is lost'.

As with any movement, waiting around to see if it works before deciding what to do next can give your opponent the fraction of a second they need to recover and do something you were not expecting.

This is not a training hall. Your attacker will not pause obligingly while you perform your next move before coming back at you with something of their own. They will be resisting you with everything they've got and either coming at you or turning, ducking or backing away from you so any delay means a lost opportunity.

So go for the knock out anyway, whether or not you go for the eyes first, and put everything you have into that blow.

Just a few more things to consider

It's worth mentioning here that a percussive strike to the jaw, while it might knock out an opponent, could also break your hand!

Now a broken hand may be preferable to a lot of alternatives we can think of. The trouble is that, if it doesn't do the job of rendering your assailant senseless, you now have an even bigger problem: you only have one hand, probably your weakest hand, to fight with.

So here's another advantage that Tai Chi can offer. By hitting with a Tai Chi punch, your fist barely travels any distance at all. There is little impact bone on bone, just a huge shock wave generated from your whole body and traveling through your hand into their head.

In some ways it's like the difference between a meteor impact and an earthquake; both are equally devastating in their own ways. Conventional blows and Tai Chi punches are both potentially devastating; the difference is that a Tai Chi punch is less likely to damage your hand.

Palm strikes

Striking the jaw with an open palm is potentially just as effective as striking with a fist, and also less likely to damage your hand, whatever style of Martial Arts you practice. Not only that, but if your fingers miss the eyes, the heel of your palm is already lined up with their jaw and you just need to release your power.

When we use words like 'release your power' we absolutely do not mean blasts of 'empty force' whatever you might have read on the subject. We are here to offer practical solutions to real-life emergencies, not any kind of mystical, esoteric powers. Your fist or palm needs to be in contact with your opponent's jaw if you want to use your fa jin.

Head Butts

A favourite technique of thugs on UK streets is to bring their head down onto yours from a height, with considerable force, if you get too close. A counter manoeuvre is to lower your own head prior to impact and then bring it up again sharply to meet theirs. In real life, this has worked effectively, not only to pre-empt the strike of an assailant but also to cause them to stagger backwards and allow the application of a Tai Chi push that ended the fight.

The Turtle

While we are on the subject of keeping it real, as we have attempted to do throughout this book, we need to mention a potential vulnerability that Tai Chi practitioners can experience.

Ironically, that vulnerability comes from suspending the Crown Point and relaxing the shoulders, two fundamentals of Tai Chi Chuan. It is this posture, the very foundation of our art, which can make us easier to knock out with a percussive blow, if we are not prepared for it.

How is this possible?

As we discussed above, a person can be knocked out by causing their head and neck to whip backwards on their shoulders. Most fighters hunker down, hunch their shoulders and withdraw their neck like a turtle into its shell. This, for them, is a weakness when delivering blows as it causes them to tense up so they are heavily reliant on their arm muscles, while a Tai Chi practitioner, being relaxed and sensitive, is able to use their whole body to respond and issue their force.

In terms of defence against an incoming blow, however, the turtles have an advantage. Once they are hunched into this protective turtle shell position, like a dog with its hackles raised, it is harder to knock them out with any kind of percussive strike because their neck is protected. It's something people do unconsciously, as you saw in our list of warning signs above.

While the turtle posture may help to protect your opponent from a percussive blow, however, the shock wave from a Tai Chi punch or palm strike may still do the job of rendering them unconscious.

However, this also raises the question of what happens if they manage to hit you with a percussive strike to the head, while you are still relaxed and upright? The likelihood is that you won't know anything about it after that.

So it's worth pointing out that if you fail to dodge or intercept an incoming blow to your head, you would be wise to become the turtle and withdraw your head, raise your shoulders and brace yourself to absorb the impact. Like everything else we have talked about here, it is no guarantee that you will remain conscious but there is a better chance of doing so than if you allow them to use your head like a punch bag on a spring.

Going Low

Of course, we appear to have been obsessed, so far, with blows to the head, mainly because they are potentially the most lethal and because they can finish a fight in seconds.

Obviously, none of the above is of any use to you if your attacker is wearing a motor cycle helmet or their arms are in the way. That's when you aim for other parts of the body that are within your reach,

194

and use everything you have. Kick shins or knees, use your elbows, get in close and shoulder them or push them over.

Get away if you can but if you can't, be like a snake and wriggle free if they try to take hold of you and if you see an opening, use it.

Multiple Attackers and other unpleasant scenarios

We can talk about all of this as if the only type of villains you are likely to meet are on their own and obligingly confronting you face to face.

The reality is that they are equally likely to sneak up on you from behind, or have an accomplice or a gang of their mates with them. They may also be carrying a gun or a knife or be under the influence of drugs that give them superhuman strength. All of these things are game changers!

As one of our teachers used to say: "Multiple attackers? One is too many!"

A possible strategy, if you are surrounded, is to go straight for one person, perhaps the leader or perhaps the weakest, and take them down so that you can get past them and run away. That presupposes that you are a fast runner!

While we hope you never find yourself in this situation, we do need to say that in the dreadful event of finding yourself on the floor being kicked by two or more people, the best you can do is to curl up into a ball and protect your face and vulnerable regions.

This is very distressing even to think about but it brings home, yet again, the importance of avoiding such situations in the first place if you possibly can!

This is why, in this book, we have spent so much time exploring possible ways of avoiding trouble by being aware, recognizing risky situations and exploring how human minds work; your own and other people's.

We have seen how some of the mental and physical qualities of Tai Chi can help by providing us with:

- An upright, alert posture;

- A calm mind that can be fully present in the moment and take a wider view, and

- A non-confrontational attitude and an ability to establish rapport in order to avoid conflict, if possible

While this may increase the probability of avoiding any kind of physically challenging incident, it is not a guarantee that this will always be possible, so we have also looked at ways of preparing ourselves for any unavoidable conflict by being alert, knowing our rights and looking at the types of challenging situations that could arise and what to do about them.

The School of Hard Knocks

We would not like to leave you with the impression that we enjoy fighting. We have spent our whole lives trying to avoid trouble and we hope that our emphasis on awareness and staying out of trouble has come across in this book as our primary focus. In writing this book, however, we have not pulled any punches with respect to the realities of physical combat. Most of the advice we have offered here has come from personal experience.

As a child growing up in the mining communities of West Yorkshire, learning to fight was not a career preference, it was a necessity for day to day survival. Hardly a day went by without people squaring off in the playground or the local pub car park and going at it with everything they had in front of a crowd of cheering and goading onlookers. Even the teachers at school were complicit, inviting boys to resolve arguments by "trading leather" in the gym; donning a pair of boxing gloves and fighting it out until (after a few bruises, split lips and injuries to pride had been sustained) the teacher called an end to it and ordered the participants to shake hands. This in a school at which one lost count of the number of beatings one received from the teaching staff themselves, with rulers, slippers, wooden sticks, headmaster's cane, gym shoes, plastic dowelling (which hurt way more than a wooden stick and made one feel sick) and any other available implement, from day one of one's entry into the educational system. A favourite technique employed by the gym teacher was the "chicken wing" in which he would make you bend over, lift your shirt and then whack your back so hard that you would run forwards in agony, looking like a chicken. A bit of "Iron Shirt Qigong", at that time, would have been very welcome!

In such an environment, you get to read the warning signs of forthcoming combat very quickly, from the look in the eyes to the growled: "Outside! Now!" Sometimes, you might even get to choose your response. Sometimes you just get to discover the effectiveness of a pre-emptive strike, as applied to your own face at an early age!

With the passage of time and the accumulation of wisdom that naturally develops through regular unsought-for practice, certain skills and instincts may be acquired. The experience of having several barrels kicked out of you is gradually transformed into the ability to survive for long enough to get a satisfactory head lock on the thug who tried to punch you, while simultaneously avoiding the creep with the knife sneaking up behind you. In this latter scenario, the availability of a mate with a snooker cue has been found to be very beneficial.

The art of the pre-emptive strike can be refined and honed within such arenas of combat. A polite invitation to "Sit the f*** down", accompanied by a well-placed slap, has prevented further unpleasantness on occasion, as has a well-aimed right cross on various other occasions.

Sometimes, a fight in which two people rip the clothes off each other's backs and draw blood can end with lots of handshakes, mutual respect and the birth of a long-lasting friendship. Others are brief encounters in which some jerk tries to make you get off a bus or get out of their village but quickly changes their mind after receiving a jab to the face and an invitation to continue the discussion outside.

Some useful experience of head-butting techniques has been gained while defending one's companions, such as the workmates who were being verbally insulted with regard to their ethnicity.

As to martial arts training, being coached by one's grandfather in back-hold Highland wrestling and attending Karate classes after school was found to be surprisingly unhelpful in real-life settings where punches and kicks did little to hamper the progress of an oncoming thug twice one's own size. Such situations did, however, give rise to an awareness of the efficacy of alternative unarmed combat strategies, only some of which are discussed in this volume.

Why, you might wonder, would someone with a background in wrestling, Karate, boxing and a youth spent navigating challenging situations, bother to learn the 'soft and gentle' art of Tai Chi?

Having read this book, you might be able to answer this question yourself. The harder something becomes, the more readily and spectacularly it will eventually snap. Weakness, on the other hand, allows bullies to dominate and prevail. But somewhere in the middle, there is that third thing; that hard to explain thing that we referred to in volume one as 'the mysterious It'. Neither soft nor hard, the springy resilience of Tai Chi is not just a physical state but also a kind of mental attitude and a shift in one's own approach to life and people that gives rise to a different kind of responsiveness in threatening situations. For some, this may arise naturally with time and maturity but, for others, the philosophy of Tai Chi can provide the catalyst for this shift in perspective.

We have noticed this as a kind of evolution during a lifetime. From early beginnings of coming off worst, through an intermediate stage of reacting to violence by becoming tougher and more menacing than the tough guy doing the attacking, something else has gradually taken the place of all of that.

After learning some Tai Chi, new ways of handling challenging situations have tended to be deployed. On one such occasion, it was discovered that the intention of a thug to apply a head butt could be thwarted without too much retaliatory aggression simply by lowering one's own head and bringing it upwards into their descending face before using a double handed Tai Chi palm strike/push to deliver them safely across a room and into the hands of the resident bouncers.

While working with some of the less socially well-adapted members of the community, there have been occasions when an individual made the decision to unsettle the blissful tranquillity of the Tai Chi class by having a go at the instructor. One went in with kicks and punches flying, only to find every blow diverted in a relaxed manner and himself swiftly pinned against the wall and advised that: "That's enough for today."

In a later incident, a rather large gentleman ran at the instructor like a battering ram, only to find himself intercepted, warded off, rolled back and deposited in a corner of the room.

These incidents, while infrequent, appear to have had the effect of making the students very attentive to their subsequent Tai Chi studies.

As we have mentioned many times elsewhere in this book, such apparent victories must never be allowed to give rise to self-congratulation, over-confidence and a willingness to take unnecessary risks. Better to give thanks for one's good fortune that the villain in question was not able to demonstrate a higher degree of proficiency in the use of unarmed combat techniques and was not, on that occasion, carrying a gun.

The danger, of course, with any kind of apparent success is that one can develop an ego that results in one's own undoing. Like cowboys on a quest to be the "fastest gun in the West", there will always be someone out there who is faster, younger, stronger, more skilled, armed with a more deadly weapon or just luckier on the day than oneself. By all means train hard, train smart and, hopefully, fight easy. Better still, avoid the need to fight at all if you possibly can and always remember that, however many steps you take on the road towards mastery, the only real mastery is mastery of one's own self and it should always involve humility. Ultimately, there is no such thing as a "master".

However, that does not mean that the quest for mastery is not worth the effort. As we have seen, actual physical contact can be fast, violent and potentially life-threatening. Any actions we take are likely to occur before we have time to think and much will depend on our unconscious reflexes; reflexes that can be trained. You may or may not have already been 'streetwise' before reading this book. You may or may not have attended a 'school of hard knocks', similar to or even worse than, the one we have described. We hope that you have not. Either way, we hope that by sharing our own experiences and those of our students with you, we have shown what Tai Chi Chuan can offer you as a method of self-defence and that we have provided insights that can increase the probability of your future survival so that you can enjoy a long and happy life.

Putting it All Together

Checklists

If you are ready to develop your skills further, here are a few checklists that can help you to focus your training:

Stay generally fit and well, if you can.

1. Take regular physical exercise including:

- Strength training with weights and resistance,

- Aerobic activity such as walking, cycling or swimming,

- High intensity interval training such as the Tabata Protocol or circuit training.

A combination of these three types of exercise can help you to maintain or improve your strength and endurance and improve your cardiovascular fitness so that you have the ability to run away or to fight without getting tired or out of breath too quickly.

2. If possible, practice getting down on the floor, rolling over and then standing up again so that you know that you are capable of getting back up onto your feet if you are knocked down.

Practice your basic skills, including:

1. Good stances

2. Suspending the Crown Point

3. Sinking and rooting

4. Using your waist

5. Using your dantien

6. Tai Chi breathing

Practice push hands

1. Single fixed step

2. Double fixed step

3. Moving step

Practice the martial applications of the movements of your hand forms, especially:

1. Ward off

2. Roll Back

3. Press

4. Push

5. Split

6. Pluck

7. Elbow strike

8. Shoulder stroke

9. Palm strikes

10. Punches

11. Low kicks

12. Drilling

Explore higher level Tai Chi skills, especially:

1. Ting jin

2. Peng jin

3. Fa jin

Stay out of trouble as much as you can by:

1. Walking with an upright, confident posture

2. Staying awake and alert

3. Avoiding being on your own on the streets at night.

4. Having your keys ready when you go out to your car or get to the door of your house.

5. Locking the doors once you are safely inside.

6. Avoiding advertising any wealth you have.

If you do find yourself in a challenging situation:

1. Control the space

2. Use a fence/wall/guard

3. Talk them down if you can

4. Do everything you can to get away

If all else fails and you have to fight:

1. Use a pre-emptive strike

2. If that doesn't work, keep going until the fight is over and you can get away.

And now…

Epilogue

Forget the Whole Thing

In a fight, whether it's in a competition or on the street, everything happens so fast that you don't have time to think. In some ways, that may be for the best. When our elderly student successfully thwarted the mugger who tried to steal her handbag in a crowded shopping centre, she instinctively turned around and punched him in the gut. Had she taken time to think about it, the mugger might well have been off with her bag long before her rational brain decided what to do about it.

As you have just seen in the previous chapter, if your pre-emptive strike is unsuccessful, a moment's hesitation is all it takes for an attacker to come right back at you. So keep it moving!

The ultimate objective of Tai Chi training is to become spontaneous.

There is a famous story, which we heard from our teacher and have read in various books, in which a school is about to be attacked by multiple assailants. Inside the school, the teacher takes a sword and performs a few moves with it in front of a student and then asks: "What do you remember?" When the student responds with: "Maybe half of it." The teacher performs a few different moves and asks again: "What do you remember now?" The student stammers: "Um…maybe …one or two moves, master." So the teacher performs a new, more elaborate series of movements. "Now what do you remember?" he demands. The student's shoulders sag in despair. "Honestly, master," he admits, "I don't remember any of it. I've forgotten it all." At that point the teacher gives the sword to the student, who goes out and single-handedly fights off all the bad guys.

This book has been all about training unconscious, spontaneous responses of the mind and body. It is not intended as a catalogue of skills and applications that you mentally scroll through in a crisis and then use to weigh up the best options against various criteria!

During your training, you may read, practice and explore these concepts as deeply and as often as you like, maybe developing new insights of your own in the process but, in a fight, let it go.

Learning every skill in this book does not guarantee your victory in every encounter, whether with a worthy opponent in an arena or an outright villain on the street, but if it improves your chances of survival by even one percent, then that could be the difference between whether or not you live to tell the tale and that has to be worth the effort of learning a martial art!

Further Reading and Helpful Links

YouTube Videos

Mike Loades, *Weapons that Made Britain, Episode 5 – Armour*, Produced by Lion Television for Channel 4 in association with the Discovery Channel, 2004.

https://www.youtube.com/watch?v=D4aMoCAypos

Real life self-protection by Geoff Thompson and Peter Consterdine

https://www.youtube.com/watch?v=Jvl9aX-ZI84

Geoff Thompson: *The Fence, Clip 1*

https://www.youtube.com/watch?v=T6OJnZG3joA

and *The Fence, Clip 2*

https://www.youtube.com/watch?v=2FGLhlakkUk

Colin Hamilton and Ben Morris, *Tai Chi Push Hands Drills (Tui Shou)*, Yiheyuan Martial Arts, 2011

https://www.youtube.com/watch?v=FnhqNtBZCGo

Tai Chi Applications - Yiheyuan Martial Arts 2013

https://www.youtube.com/watch?v=WPvOjVhxVPU

Articles

Marked for Mayhem, Chuck Hustmyre and Jay Dixit, Psychology Today, 2013. First Published January 1 2009

https://www.psychologytoday.com/articles/200901/marked-mayhem

Ready for anything: The best strategies to survive a disaster, (Online edition) Michael Bond. New Scientist, 10th May 2017.

https://www.newscientist.com/article/mg23431250-400-ready-for-anything-the-best-strategy-to-survive-a-disaster/

How to Survive a Disaster. Michael Bond. BBC Future.

http://www.bbc.com/future/story/20150128-how-to-survive-a-disaster

Research Papers

Attracting Assault: Victims' Nonverbal Cues. Betty Grayson and Morris I. Stein, Journal of Communication, Volume 31, Issue 1, pages 68-75, March 1981

http://onlinelibrary.wiley.com/doi/10.1111/j.1460-2466.1981.tb01206.x/full

Good Samaritanism: An Underground Phenomenon? Piliavin, Irving M.; Rodin, Judith; Piliavin, Jane A. Journal of Psychology, Volume 13(4), December 1969, pp289-299

Books

Tai Chi Classics, Waysun Liao, Shambhala, 1977. ISBN 0-87773-531-X. New Edition 2001. ISBN-10: 1570627495, ISBN-13: 978-1570627491

Taijiquan: Die Tradition der 13 Grundformen, Professor Wang Zhizhong, Shaker Media, 2014. Translated from Chinese into German by Gudrun Gerbstedt. ISBN-10: 3-95631-126-4 /3956311264, ISBN-13: 978-3-95631-126-0 /9783956311260

Tai Ji Jin: Discoveries on Intrinsic Energies for Mastery of Self-Defense Skills, (Volume 2 of a translation of the Private Family Records of Master Yang Luchan), Stuart Alve Olson, Valley Spirit Arts, Phoenix, Arizona, 2013

Advanced Yang Style Tai Chi Chuan Volumes 1 and 2, Dr. Yang, Jwing Ming, Yang's Martial Arts Association, 1986 Republished as: *Tai Chi Chuan Martial Power: Advanced Yang Style.* YMAA Publication Center; 3rd revised edition 16 April 2015. ISBN-10: 1594392943, ISBN-13: 978-1594392948

Armed Robbers in Action: Stickups and Street Culture. Richard T. Wright and Scott H. Decker. Northeastern Series in Criminal Behaviour, University Press of New England, 1997. ISBN-13: 978-1-55553-784-5 (e-book)

The Psychopath Test: A Journey through the Madness Industry, Jon Ronson, Picador, 2011. ISBN: 978-1-4472-0250-9 EPUB

Finish a Fight in One Move: Without Any Training, Justyn Billingham, 2015.

Tai Chi Touchstones: Yang Family Secret Transmissions, Douglas Wile, Sweet Ch'i Press, 1983. ISBN-10: 091205901X, ISBN-13: 978-0912059013

Lost T'ai-chi Classics from the Late Ch'ing Dynasty, Douglas Wile, Albany: SUNY, 1996. ISBN-10: 0791426548, ISBN-13: 978-0791426548

Translations Online

Methods of Applying Taiji Boxing. Dong Huling, 1956. Translated by Paul Brennan

https://brennantranslation.wordpress.com/2017/01/27/dong-hulings-applications/

(There are many other translations of excellent works on this site – well worth a visit!)

T'ai Chi Ch'uan classics (All the main Tai Chi classics, as researched and interpreted by Lee N. Scheele)

http://www.scheele.org/lee/classics.html

Martial Arts Organisations and Governing Bodies

The British Council for Chinese Martial Arts (BCCMA)

https://bccma.com/

The Tai Chi Union for Great Britain (TCUGB)

http://www.taichiunion.com/

The British Combat Association (BCA) Established by Peter Consterdine and Geoff Thompson

http://britishcombat.co.uk/index.aspx

The British Self Defence Governing Body. The Centre for Physical Interventions. Incorporated under authority of Statutory Instrument 1685

http://www.bsdgb.co.uk/index.php?Information:Law_Relating_to_S elf_Defence

Legal Right to Use Force

Self Defence and the Prevention of Crime. Legal Guidance from the Crown Prosecution Service

http://www.cps.gov.uk/legal/s_to_u/self_defence/#Reasonable_Forc e

U.K. Statistics on Violence

Violence at work: Findings from the Crime Survey for England and Wales and the Reporting of Injuries, Diseases and Dangerous Occurrences and Regulations. *The Health and Safety at Work Executive.* 2015/16.

http://www.hse.gov.uk/statistics/causinj/violence/index.htm

Overview of Violent Crime and Sexual Offences. *Office for National Statistics,* March 2016

By the Authors

Companion Volume in the 7 Steps Towards Mastery Series

How to Move Towards Tai Chi Mastery: 7 Practical Steps to Improve your Forms and Access your Internal Power, Colin and Gaynel Hamilton, 2018. ISBN: 9781980688921

Magazine Articles

Hamilton, G., *Britain's Best Kept Secret?: An Interview with Master Zhu,* Tai Chi Chuan Magazine: The Journal of the Tai Chi Union for Great Britain, Issue 10, pages 38-41, 1998.

A Circular Route to Tai Chi Mastery, Hamilton, G., Tai Chi Chuan and Oriental Arts Magazine: The Journal of the Tai Chi Union for Great Britain, Issue 49, pages 24-26, 2015

There Are No Secrets? Well, Actually..., Hamilton, G., Tai Chi Chuan and Oriental Arts Magazine: The Journal of the Tai Chi Union for Great Britain, Issue 50, pages 44-45, 2016

Free eBooks for beginners (as downloadable pdf files):

Hamilton, G., *Your Tai Chi Companion Part 1: Getting Started.* Yiheyuan Martial Arts, 2009. www.taichileeds.com

Hamilton, G., *Your Tai Chi Companion Part 2: Moving On.* Yiheyuan Martial Arts, 2012. www.taichileeds.com

Made in the USA
Lexington, KY
16 May 2018